Mind-Body Medicine: The New Science of Optimal Health

Jason M. Satterfield, Ph.D.

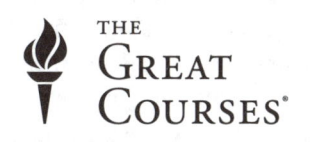

THE
GREAT
COURSES®

PUBLISHED BY:

THE GREAT COURSES
Corporate Headquarters
4840 Westfields Boulevard, Suite 500
Chantilly, Virginia 20151-2299
Phone: 1-800-832-2412
Fax: 703-378-3819
www.thegreatcourses.com

Copyright © The Teaching Company, 2013

Printed in the United States of America

This book is in copyright. All rights reserved.

Without limiting the rights under copyright reserved above,
no part of this publication may be reproduced, stored in
or introduced into a retrieval system, or transmitted,
in any form, or by any means
(electronic, mechanical, photocopying, recording, or otherwise),
without the prior written permission of
The Teaching Company.

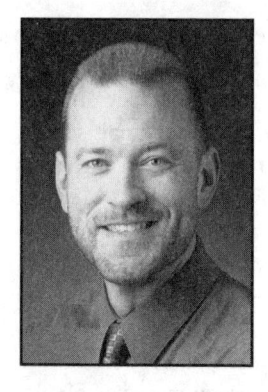

Jason M. Satterfield, Ph.D.

Professor of Clinical Medicine
University of California, San Francisco

Professor Jason M. Satterfield is Professor of Clinical Medicine, Director of Social and Behavioral Sciences, and Director of Behavioral Medicine in the Division of General Internal Medicine at the University of California, San Francisco (UCSF). He received his B.S. in Brain Sciences from the Massachusetts Institute of Technology with a special minor in Psychology from Harvard University. He completed his Ph.D. in Clinical Psychology at the University of Pennsylvania (Penn), where he worked with Dr. Martin Seligman on cognitive models of bias, risk taking, depression, and aggression. Professor Satterfield was trained as a cognitive-behavioral therapist at Penn's Center for Cognitive Therapy under the supervision of Drs. Aaron T. Beck, Judith Beck, and Robert DeRubeis. Professor Satterfield completed his internship and postdoctoral fellowship at UCSF at San Francisco General Hospital with Drs. Ricardo Muñoz, Jeanne Miranda, and Jacqueline Persons in the Department of Psychiatry. In 1996, Professor Satterfield accepted a position in the UCSF Division of General Internal Medicine to focus on the intersection of psychological factors and physical health.

Professor Satterfield's clinical work has included adaptations to cognitive-behavioral therapy groups for underserved, medically ill populations and psychological interventions for patients at the beginning of the end of life. He currently directs the UCSF Behavioral Medicine Unit, which integrates mental and behavioral health services into adult primary care.

Professor Satterfield's research and educational interests include integrating behavioral science in medical education, disseminating and implementing evidence-based behavioral practices, and developing educational strategies to address health-care disparities. His current projects include promoting physician social and emotional intelligence, constructing integrated behavioral health models for primary care, developing screening and brief interventions for substance abuse, and integrating the social and behavioral sciences in medical school and medical residency curricula. Professor Satterfield is a member of the Behavioral and Social Science Consortium for Medical Education and the Council for Training in Evidence-Based Behavioral Practice, both of which are funded by the National Institutes of Health.

Professor Satterfield's book *A Cognitive-Behavioral Approach to the Beginning of the End of Life: Minding the Body* was recognized as a Self-Help Book of Merit by the Association for Behavioral and Cognitive Therapies. His special clinical publications include treatment models for group psychotherapy, treatment adaptations to improve cultural competence, and a transdisciplinary model to promote evidence-based behavioral practices in medicine, including interventions for smoking, weight management, drug abuse, and chronic disease management. Professor Satterfield is coauthor of a recent report detailing the role of behavioral science in medicine, and he served on the Behavioral and Social Science Subcommittee that revised the Medical College Admission Test (MCAT)—work that was recently featured in the *New England Journal of Medicine* and *The New York Times*. Professor Satterfield is also part of a core interdisciplinary team that is writing a medical textbook based on the biopsychosocial model.

Professor Satterfield currently directs the Social and Behavioral Sciences curriculum for all UCSF medical students and internal medicine. He has been nominated for multiple teaching awards at UCSF, including the Robert H. Crede Award for Excellence in Teaching, the Kaiser Award for Excellence in Teaching, and the Academy of Medical Educators Cooke Award for the Scholarship of Teaching and Learning. He is often competitively selected to teach at national conferences for a wide variety of health professionals, including physicians, nurses, social workers, and psychologists.

Professor Satterfield grew up in Middle Tennessee and was the first in his family to attend college. After living in Boston and Philadelphia for school, he moved in 1994 to San Francisco. He is an avid traveler and enjoys a large circle of friends and family. ∎

Table of Contents

INTRODUCTION

Professor Biography i
Course Scope 1

LECTURE GUIDES

LECTURE 1
Weaving the Biopsychosocial Braid 3

LECTURE 2
Vital Signs—Defining Health and Illness 9

LECTURE 3
Fight or Flight vs. Rest and Digest 15

LECTURE 4
Simmering Soup—The Neuroendocrine System 22

LECTURE 5
Deploying the Troops—Basic Immunology 28

LECTURE 6
Nature vs. Nurture—Genes, Health, and Disease 35

LECTURE 7
Forget Me Not—Cognitive Function 41

LECTURE 8
Mind over Matter—Cognition in Everyday Life 47

LECTURE 9
Emotions Revealed—Psychology of Emotions 53

LECTURE 10
Agony and Ecstasy—Biology of Emotion 59

Table of Contents

LECTURE 11
What's Your EQ, and How Can You Improve It? 66

LECTURE 12
What's Your Type? Personality and Health 73

LECTURE 13
An Apple a Day—Behavior and Disease Prevention........80

LECTURE 14
Staying on the Wagon—Making Changes That Last.......86

LECTURE 15
Ease the Burn—Modern-Day Stress and Coping............92

LECTURE 16
The Iceberg—Visible and Hidden Identity 99

LECTURE 17
Ties That Bind—Relationships and Health 106

LECTURE 18
Building Bridges—Intimacy and Relationships 113

LECTURE 19
Touched by Grace—Spirituality and Health...................120

LECTURE 20
A Matter of Class—Socioeconomics and Health 127

LECTURE 21
A Cog in the Wheel—Occupational Stress 134

LECTURE 22
The Power of Place—Communities and Health 141

LECTURE 23
The Master Plan—Public Health and Policy..................148

Table of Contents

LECTURE 24
Heart and Soul—Cardiovascular Disease I 154

LECTURE 25
Heart and Soul—Cardiovascular Disease II 160

LECTURE 26
The Big C—Cancer and Mind-Body Medicine 167

LECTURE 27
Bugs, Drugs, and Buddha—Psychoneuroimmunology 174

LECTURE 28
Fire in the Belly—The GI System 180

LECTURE 29
Obesity—America's New Epidemic 187

LECTURE 30
The Strain in Pain Lies Mainly in the Brain 194

LECTURE 31
Catching Your Zs—Sleep and Health 201

LECTURE 32
Chasing Zebras—Somatoform Disorders 207

LECTURE 33
Seeing the Glass Half Empty—Depression 214

LECTURE 34
Silencing the Scream—Understanding Anxiety 221

LECTURE 35
Lingering Wounds—Trauma, Resilience, Growth 228

LECTURE 36
Tomorrow's Biopsychosocial Medicine 234

Table of Contents

SUPPLEMENTAL MATERIAL

Bibliography..241

Disclaimer

These lectures are not designed for use as medical references to diagnose, treat, or prevent medical illnesses or trauma. Neither The Great Courses nor Professor Jason Satterfield is responsible for your use of this educational material or its consequences. If you have questions about the diagnosis, treatment, or prevention of a medical condition or illness, you should consult a qualified physician.

Mind-Body Medicine: The New Science of Optimal Health

Scope:

In less than half a century, medicine has gone from dismissing holistic approaches to health to actively studying and, in some cases, practicing mind-body medicine. Few would disagree that stress and emotion affect our health in sometimes profound and important ways. However, a truly holistic approach is even broader still. It includes emotions and stress but also recognizes how our social environments, relationships, and beliefs are related to health and disease.

This course explores the history, development, and evidence base for an approach called biopsychosocial medicine, in which biology, psychology, and sociocultural factors are examined as both independent and interactive contributors to health and disease. This conceptual model is first introduced, followed by essential biomedical building blocks, an exploration of psychological and sociological variables, and, finally, applications to organ systems and common chronic diseases. This course draws from diverse research traditions, poignant clinical narratives, and active demonstrations compiled from nearly 20 years of educational training programs in medicine, nursing, psychology, and anthropology.

This course seeks to answer three key questions: What makes us sick? What makes us well? What can we do about it? By exploring both biological as well as psychosocial factors related to health, you will graduate with a cutting-edge understanding of how the "outside" (e.g., stress, relationships, work) gets "inside" to alter the functioning of our minds and bodies. And, more importantly, you will finish this course with a toolbox of ideas and interventions useful in pursuing your personal health goals.

This course is organized into five interdependent sections: Introduction, Biological Pathways, Psychological Factors, Social Factors, and Diseases. In the first section (Introduction), the course begins by defining the biopsychosocial model, its emergence, and its current applications in modern medicine. The lectures in the first section attempt to define the health of individuals, families, and communities to assist you in doing your own health assessments.

The second section (Biological Pathways) covers basic and fundamental biomedical pathways that help you understand "how the outside gets inside." These four pathways include the autonomic nervous system, the neuroendocrine system, immunology, and genetics.

The third section (Psychological Factors) examines the evidence supporting links between cognition, emotions, personality, behavior, stress, and health. You will learn why we often engage in unhealthy behaviors and why behavior changes can be so difficult to make. You will have the opportunity to perform a number of psychological and behavioral self-assessments while critically appraising the promise of psychological interventions on health and behavior change.

The fourth section (Social Factors) analyzes social and ecological factors that are thought to be critical to health and disease. These factors include identity, culture, socioeconomic status, social support, occupational stress, and public health.

The fifth and final section (Diseases) uses the three "braids" of the biopsychosocial model to help you understand causes, consequences, and treatments of common chronic diseases, such as cardiovascular disease, cancer, obesity, chronic pain, insomnia, depression, anxiety, and post-traumatic stress disorder.

Upon completion of this course, you will have a more complete and nuanced scientific understanding of what makes us sick, what makes us well, and what we can do about it. You will have a greater appreciation of the roles of the individual, family, community, and society in promoting health—in its most narrow and broadest definitions. And, lastly, you will have more insight into how our current, mostly biological medical system works, including where it excels and where it fails. When armed with this new insight and information, savvy patients and consumers may more effectively partner with their medical provider and maximize their health. ■

Weaving the Biopsychosocial Braid
Lecture 1

Throughout this course, the goal is to answer three key questions: Why do people get sick? How do people get well? What can we do about it? As you proceed through the course, it is important to have great concentration and great compassion—great concentration in being able to synthesize, understand, and apply the science from the many different disciplines that you will learn about and great compassion in being able to experience, feel, and connect to many of the clinical stories that you are going to be exposed to. The goal is to learn from and apply those stories to yourself and to your loved ones.

The Baby Monica Study

- A paradigm of health, the biopsychosocial model helps us understand the relationship between biological factors, psychological factors, and social factors. It helps us understand how the outside gets inside—how stress, environment, jobs, and families affect the way that our body functions biologically.

- The originator of the biopsychosocial model, George Engel, might attribute the model to a one-year-old baby girl named Monica.

- In the baby Monica study, psychiatrists examined this one-year-old girl who had been born with a congenital condition called esophageal atresia, which means that she was born with an esophagus that didn't properly connect to the stomach. It often requires several surgeries but can be fixed and isn't considered fatal.

- When Monica was in the hospital, she had a stomach tube that was placed so that her nurses—her caregivers—could feed her directly through the stomach tube.

- The idea of the experiment was as follows: The psychiatrist would play the friendly doctor, developing a relationship with Monica so that she would feel comfortable around him. George Engel would be the unfriendly, scary stranger so that she would be afraid of him.

- Because the psychiatrists had direct access to her stomach, they could directly measure gastric secretions. Whenever the "friendly" psychiatrist would come into the room, baby Monica was happy and excited, and her digestive juices were flowing. Whenever Engel would walk into the room, she was afraid and would sometimes cry and withdraw, and her gastric secretions would stop.

- Although Engel might not call this a eureka moment, it was certainly formative in terms of shaping his thinking about the biopsychosocial model. It wasn't until about 20 years later that he coined the term "biopsychosocial model" in his paper that came out in *Science* magazine, and since then, he has trained scores of health professionals in the biopsychosocial model and how to apply it to medical care.

Pop Quiz: Mind-Body Connections
- **True or false: The day before enduring a midterm exam, the average student will have significant increases in systolic blood pressure.** This statement is true. In fact, it has been proven so many times that it's not even considered terribly interesting anymore.

- **True or false: High occupational stress can double your risk of dying from cardiovascular disease.** This statement is true. Since a study published in the *British Medical Journal* in 2002, there have been a number of systematic reviews that summarize over a dozen different studies showing that occupational stress is bad for your heart.

- **True or false: People who average less than seven hours of sleep per night have triple the risk of catching a cold compared to people who average eight hours or more sleep per night.** This statement is true. This is the work of Sheldon Cohen, published in 2009 in the *Archives of Internal Medicine*.

Neuroanatomy

- When learning about neuroanatomy, it's helpful to pull out an old concept called the triune brain, which was first written about by Paul MacLean in the 1920s/1930s. The triune brain is the idea that the brain is divided into three parts that are based on how old they are evolutionarily but also on when they develop in terms of human development.

- The oldest parts of our brain are toward the rear and lower down our brain stem—our cerebellum, for instance. This is also called the reptilian brain; it's the more primitive brain from an evolutionary sense.

- Higher up is the mammalian brain. If you imagine looking through to the center of the brain, this is our limbic system, which is responsible for much of our emotional life—at least the primitive emotional motivations.

To understand mind-body medicine, we have to understand the mind; in order to understand the mind, we have to understand the brain.

- The highest level of the brain is the human brain. The highest level of functioning takes place in our frontal lobes, which in humans are about a third of our brains—much more than we see in any other animals. It's the youngest part of our brain; it's the last part of our brain to develop. In fact, our frontal lobes don't develop until we're approximately 25 years old.

- Neurons are the primary cells that are within our brains. We have about 100 billion neurons in our brains and about 7,000 connections for each of those neurons. This means that we have about 700 trillion connections within our brain. Somehow, seemingly magically, it's that firing and that interconnectedness that gives rise to the mind.

- The neurons communicate with one another through neurotransmitters, such as serotonin, norepinephrine, and dopamine. Neurons actually comprise only 15 percent of our brain cells. The rest are glial cells, or supportive cells.

Brain Myths
- **Myth: We only use about 10 percent of our brain.** This myth has been around for decades. We actually use all of our brain. All of the levels of the triune brain interact and talk to one another, although they may be active or inactive at a particular time.

- **Myth: We only have one set learning style.** Educational psychologists for decades have been trying to test out the idea of visual versus auditory versus kinesthetic learners, and they found that people do indeed have preferences. However, if a person is put in an experiment, he or she can learn things just as well by reading, listening, or doing. Research has shown that if you want to be the most effective learner, multimodal learning helps the most.

- **Myth: We have a separation between our left and right brain. (Our left brain is the rational brain, and the right brain is the creative brain.)** While it is true that there are certain localized functions—such as language is more commonly seen on the left side of the brain—both sides of our brain are in close coordination with one another. Creative activities can stimulate the left brain; rational activities can stimulate the right brain.

The Mind
- Think of the brain as the hardware that gives rise to the software, which is the mind—a software that in essence writes itself and adapts itself and is always changing.

- Our brains gives rise to our mind. Our mind includes consciousness, learning, identity, and life experiences—the sum total of who we are. It's those interpretations of brain function that we want to understand because that's what influences our body and our health.

Pop Quiz: Health-Related Behaviors
- **What percentage of patients are nonadherent to their antihypertensive medication (blood pressure pills)?** The answer is about 50 percent.

- **How many people in the United States have or will have an alcohol or drug addiction?** The percentage is about 10 percent, which equates to over 20 million people.

- **Behavior accounts for what percentage of premature mortality?** That answer is about 40 to 50 percent. The amount of our health-care budget that is spent on behavior—5 percent—is certainly not proportional to the degree that behavior contributes to premature mortality.

Pop Quiz: Social and Cultural Contributors to Health
- **African American men, ages 55 to 64, are how much more likely to die from stroke or diabetes compared to Caucasian American men their age?** The answer is that African American men have triple the risk.

- **True or false: Single men die sooner than married men, but single women live as long or longer than married women.** This statement is true. In fact, research shows that the increased risk of single men dying prematurely is about 32 percent higher than married men.

- **True or false: In the United States, 1 in 10 people has limited English proficiency and over 20 percent of households speak a language other than English.** This statement is true. We live in a diverse country that is growing more and more diverse year after year. It would behoove us to understand how we can best care for people of all different languages and cultural backgrounds.

The Biopsychosocial Model
- Just as behavioral factors play a critical role in our health, so do social factors, including education, income, family, culture, race,

gender, and sexuality. Even if you look at what might be considered one of the most biomedical causes of disease—genetics—there are still social factors.

- Heredity may put us at risk for disease, essentially giving us limitations, but within that range, social and behavioral factors may make us more or less likely to get sick or to stay well.

- In the biopsychosocial model, these three strands—the biological, the psychological, and the social—are woven together. As you proceed through this course, as the course starts to tackle common chronic diseases that many of us are currently experiencing or will experience at some point in the future, always ask yourself what the biological, psychological, and social factors are.

Suggested Reading

Breedlove, Watson, and Rosenzsweig, *Biological Psychology*.

Engel, "The Clinical Application of the Biopsychosocial Model."

———, "The Need for a New Medical Model."

Engel, "George L. Engel, M.D., 1913–1999."

Johnson, *Mind Wide Open*.

Questions to Consider

1. All animals have brains, but do they have "minds"? What does it take to cross the threshold from brain to mind?

2. If behavioral and social determinants of health are so important, why do we spend such little time teaching about them or using them to improve health?

Vital Signs—Defining Health and Illness
Lecture 2

What does it mean to be healthy? In this lecture, you will learn about the multidimensionality of health. You will examine some basic epidemiologic data—some of the leading causes of death; how these have changed over time; and how different biological, psychological, and social factors matter. You will be introduced to infant mortality and health disparities. Hopefully, by the end of this lecture, you will move to a more holistic view of health that doesn't focus on the absence or presence of disease.

Theories of Health

- In terms of our underlying, implicit theories of health—or, specifically, what causes us to be healthy or what causes us to be sick—our current thinking is primarily dominated by the idea of pathogenesis: of how pathology or how diseases are generated. Primarily, we know that diseases are generated via germ theory, which involves looking at microbes, viruses, and bacteria.

- This, of course, is better than some of the historical alternatives, which were that we thought diseases were caused by possession by demons, by soul loss, by getting the evil eye, and by taboo violations.

- Even in modern times, there are a number of different cultural variations to the germ theory, including Eastern medicine. For example, traditional Chinese medicine involves looking at the balance of hot and cold or looking at the flow of Chi, or energy, throughout the meridians of the body.

- The biopsychosocial model should not necessarily be thought of as a theory of health; instead, it should be thought of as a grander organizing theory that can pull in different culturally bound beliefs to help us understand the biological, psychological, and social contributions to what makes us healthy, what makes us sick, and what we can do about it.

Defining and Measuring Health

- The word "health" comes from an old English word that means "being whole, sound, or well." Standard medical dictionaries define the term as "the state of the organism when it functions optimally without evidence of disease or abnormality."

- Instead of trying to define it, think about health as a multidimensional, complex construct that includes the body and biology but also the mind, spirit, relationships, community, and maybe even society.

- One way to measure health is by the presence or absence of disease. We have all sorts of ways to test whether you have heart disease or diabetes, for example. Measuring health, though, might also involve physical fitness, mental health, or social or behavioral aspects of health. It could involve quality of life, satisfaction, or optimal functioning.

- The most common way that we measure health is through your yearly visit to your primary care doctor. Depending on your age, you may have a whole host of different sorts of screening tests to rule out different diseases.

- If you're interested in being psychologically healthy or assessing your psychological health, you might go to see a psychologist, who would give you a Structured Clinical Interview for the DSM (SCID). The DSM (Diagnostic and Statistical Manual of Mental Disorders) is the diagnostic bible for mental illnesses.

- If you look at the health of an individual in many research studies, they use a self-report measure called the SF-36. This is the short-form health survey that was originally a much longer survey from a study done by the RAND Corporation, which identified eight dimensions of health: vitality, physical functioning, bodily pain, general health perceptions, physical role functioning, emotional role functioning, social role functioning, and mental health.

- This is all about self-reporting, so we don't have information on whether or not an individual has some of the precursors of disease. If we want a more complete, holistic view of health, we might combine something like the SF-36 with that yearly visit to a primary care doctor.

- Some of the most commonly used measures of health in populations are mortality rates: Who dies? When do they die? What do they die of?

- One of the bellwether measures of the health of a nation is infant mortality, which is defined as when an infant dies before one year of age. It is reported as a ratio of deaths per 1,000 births.

- Another mortality measure is life expectancy. In the United States, life expectancy for women is 81 years while expectancy for men is 76 years. This statistic varies by race, socioeconomic status, and geography.

- The country with the best life expectancy is Japan, where life expectancy is 86 for women and 79 for men. The United States is ranked 38th in the world in terms of life expectancy.

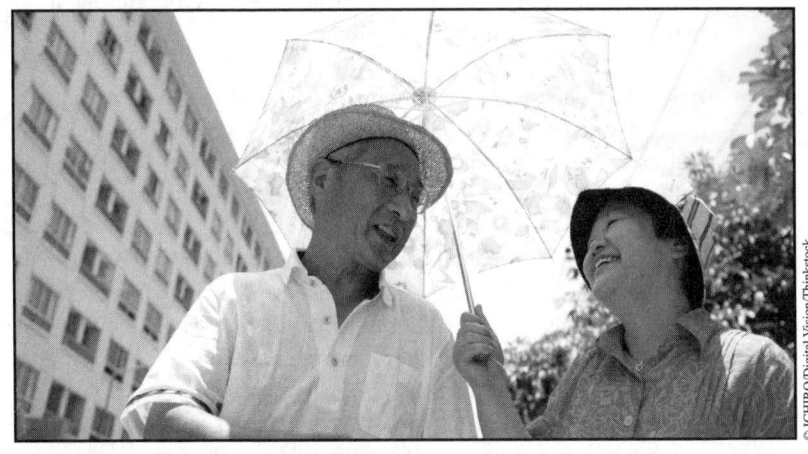

Health doesn't just have to be about the absence of disease. It can be about the quality of life, mental health, spirituality, and relationships.

Determinants of Health

- The cause of death has dramatically changed over the past 100 years or so. The leading causes of death about 100 years ago were acute infectious illnesses, such as influenza, pneumonia, and tuberculosis. In modern times, the leading causes of death, by far, are heart disease and cancer. These are chronic diseases; they don't have a sudden onset.

- In fact, these diseases have a very strong behavioral component, which is why the biopsychosocial model—understanding behavior and psychology—has become so important.

- This has important implications for health-care providers but also for us. The knowledge base and skill set of a health-care provider needs to change: It's not about prevention or treatment of acute infectious illnesses; it's about prevention and treatment of chronic diseases.

- For patients who are at risk for developing those chronic diseases—and most of us will eventually develop them—it behooves us to understand how we can slow them, how we can manage them, and how we can work with our health-care team to prolong our lives both in terms of quality and quantity.

- Behavior accounts for approximately 40 percent of premature mortality. Genetics accounts for about 30 percent while social factors account for about 15 percent. The environment accounts for only 5 percent, and health care accounts for only 10 percent.

- Together, behavior and social factors account for about 55 percent of premature mortality. We're currently spending about 5 percent of health-care dollars on behavioral interventions, despite the fact that they account for 55 percent of premature mortality.

- It might be time to rethink the way we train our physicians and the way we provide medicine. If we break down the list of behaviors into specific behaviors, tobacco has the greatest contribution to premature mortality—by far. Smoking cigarettes is accountable for about 19 to 20 percent of premature mortality. Second is diet and then activity patterns (and, of course, its relationship to obesity and diabetes and a number of other diseases). Alcohol, microbial agents, and toxic agents come after that.

- The World Health Organization has a list of six determinants for health other than behavior: geography, environment, genetics, income, education level, and relationships.

- It is due to these and other determinants of health that we see health disparities in disease prevalence and outcomes in different populations.

- For example, in the state of California, African Americans have a 61 percent higher age-adjusted mortality rate than Caucasian Americans. In addition, Mexican Americans are 200 percent more likely to develop diabetes compared to Caucasian Americans, and Vietnamese women are five times more likely to develop cervical cancer compared to Caucasian women.

- These health disparities could be due to biological reasons or genetic differences or psychological variables, but it's probably about a mixture of all of these things. Of course, we want to find an answer because hopefully we want to do something about it. To do so, we need to move to a more holistic paradigm of health.

Public Health Initiatives
- There are a few broad public health initiatives that have stimulated a lot of thought, discussion, and hopefully some changes in our health-care system—as well as activating patients to be more active collaborators in their health care.

- The Healthy People Initiative was launched by the Department of Health and Human Services in 1979 as a systematic approach to health improvement. They set goals and baseline targets every 10 years.

- The 2010 plan focused on two overarching goals: increasing the quality of life (including the years of healthy life) and eliminating health disparities. There were 28 focus areas and 467 measurable outcomes. Life expectancy has increased by a few percentage points, but unfortunately, health disparities—including smoking and obesity—have actually gotten worse.

- Healthy People 2020 has four overarching goals: quality of life, healthy development, healthy behaviors across the life span, and a focus on the social and physical environments that promote health. In Healthy People 2020, there are 42 topic areas, 600 objectives, and 1,200 measures. Fortunately, they've pulled out 26 leading health indicators that are organized into 12 topic areas.

- Visit healthypeople.gov if you're interested in learning more about the leading health indicators and what you can do so that you and your family are pushing yourself closer toward optimal states of health.

Suggested Reading

Becker, Glascoff, and Felts, "Salutogenesis 30 Years Later."

McGinnis, Ruso, and Knickman. "The Case for More Active Policy Attention to Health Promotion."

Questions to Consider

1. If health is more than the absence of disease, what else does it include? How could you measure it?

2. Using the broader definition of "health," should the health-care system remain primarily focused on disease and leave "health" to others? Who would those "others" be?

Fight or Flight vs. Rest and Digest
Lecture 3

This lecture will give you an overview of the autonomic nervous system. You will learn about the basic anatomy and physiology—the form and function—of the autonomic nervous system. Specifically, you will learn about the fight-or-flight response and about the stress-response system. In addition, you will be exposed to some specific examples of diseases that are related to either overactivity or underactivity of the autonomic nervous system. As you go about your day, think about events that may trigger your autonomic nervous system.

The Autonomic Nervous System: Form

- The nervous system can be divided into the central nervous system (CNS) and the peripheral nervous system (PNS). The CNS is composed of the brain and the spinal cord.

- The PNS can be divided further into the autonomic nervous system and the somatic nervous system. The somatic nervous system is responsible for the voluntary control of our muscles. The autonomic nervous system is mostly about stimulation, but the one exception is digestion.

- The autonomic nervous system is called "autonomic" for a few different reasons. Originally, people thought that it was autonomous from the central nervous system—but that's absolutely not true. It's also called "autonomic" because it's automatic. It innervates most of our internal organs. Breathing, the act of your heart beating, and digestion happen automatically and in response to our environment, which might cause us to be more activated or deactivated.

- The autonomic nervous system also divides into two branches: the sympathetic nervous system and the parasympathetic nervous system. The sympathetic nervous system is responsible primarily for turning things up, and the parasympathetic nervous system is responsible primarily for turning things down.

- In terms of anatomy and physiology—form and function—there are general visceral motor and sensory neurons as part of the autonomic nervous system. They are both afferent and efferent. Afferent means that it goes from the body to the brain while efferent means that it goes from the brain to the body.

- The autonomic nervous system can be either excitatory, turning things up, or inhibitory, turning things down. The sensory input that we receive from our body is almost always unconscious, but sometimes it is not. If we have pain in our internal organs, we can often feel it. Other sensations, such as the sensation of satiety, we might not be fully aware of.

- Where does all of this knowledge about autonomics come from? Originally, it comes from the work of Walter Cannon. Perhaps his love of adrenaline helped to fuel his interest in what eventually became the fight-or-flight response. In 1915, as Chair of Psychology at Harvard, he coined the term "fight or flight."

- Since then, we've added a third "f" to that equation: fight, flight, or freeze. We know that some animals, including humans at times, have a defensive response to freeze, presumably because some predators' visual systems are activated when they see movement or motion. If we are immobile, then maybe that will keep us safe.

- Much of Cannon's work was popularized in his 1932 book called *The Wisdom of the Body*, in which he talked about the fight-or-flight response—which was initially studied in rats, then in monkeys, and then of course in humans.

- The other important idea that Cannon introduced is the idea of homeostasis, which is the idea that we want to keep things balanced. We have a particular baseline that is healthiest for us, and we want to do what we can to try to stay at that baseline. Unfortunately, life knocks us off balance.

- Cannon talked about different systems in the body that try to pull us back to homeostasis. For example, he talked about blood sugar: We eat, and our blood sugar goes up; then, our insulin, which we secrete, pulls our blood sugar back down. In addition, our body temperature, depending on the ambient temperature and on our level of activity, may go up or down. If we are hot, we sweat to cool us off. If we are cold, we shiver so that our muscles are more active, raising our body temperature. Cannon thought that the autonomic nervous system operated in approximately the same way.

The Autonomic Nervous System: Function

- There is a set of chemical messengers that are used in order for the autonomic nervous system to be able to communicate with itself and with its target organs. The two chemicals that are most commonly used are norepinephrine and epinephrine, which are also known as noradrenaline and adrenaline, respectively.

- These chemicals can be released either as neurotransmitters or as hormones. Whether it's a neurotransmitter or hormone has nothing to do with the structure of the molecule; it depends on where and how it's released.

- If it is a neurotransmitter, it means that it is released from the axon of one neuron and picked up by the dendrites of another neuron—a very small distance and a very precise and quick form of communication. If it is a hormone, it's usually released directly into the bloodstream, so it circulates freely throughout the body. It takes longer for it to turn things on, and it also takes longer to turn off. The process is a little bit messier, but the effects can be distributed throughout the body—not just from one neuron to the next neuron.

- Adrenaline is primarily responsible for the fight-or-flight response. That adrenaline surge is called cardiovascular reactivity. Essentially, our cardiovascular system is responsible for pumping blood, energy, nutrients, and oxygen to help our body to function.

- Our cardiovascular reactivity is responsible for helping us to be able to meet those threats that are ahead of us: Our blood pressure and heart rate go up; and we have either vasodilation, where our arteries open wider to allow more blood to flow, or we have vasoconstriction.

- When you're in a fight-or-flight response, there is a complex chain in which the blood is preferentially sent throughout your body. You want the oxygen and energy to go to your heart as well as to your arms and legs so that you can fight or flee.

- You need energy, which means that you're going to need some blood sugar. Activating the autonomic nervous system, particularly the sympathetic nervous system, increases your level of blood sugar. It also increases your attention and your focus, but it gives you a sort of tunnel vision, presumably to help you focus on whatever danger might lie ahead of you to help you escape it.

Fight-or-Flight Response: Individual Variability
- There's a fair amount of individual variability in terms of how robust or how sensitive we are to the adrenaline-soaked fight-or-flight response. Of course, there are going to be some biological differences, probably due to genetics. However, remember the biopsychosocial model, including psychological and social factors.

- We know from animal studies as well as human studies that early life experiences can actually retrain and, in fact, sensitize our autonomic nervous system. If you've learned that your environment is hostile, it would behoove you to have a supersensitive trigger so that you can quickly and robustly respond to those dangers that happen to be frequently in your environment.

- In addition, we know that people that have experienced intense traumas may develop posttraumatic stress disorder, and as part of this disorder, we see increased sympathetic nervous system arousal as well as an arousal of the hypothalamic-pituitary-adrenal (HPA) axis part of the stress-response system.

- Given the changes in sensitivity, given the responsiveness to our environment—to early life events and maybe to traumas later in life—we can train or retrain our autonomic nervous system. In fact, training of the autonomic nervous system is a normal part of life. For example, as children, we train ourselves to use the bathroom at socially appropriate times.

Stress
- Stress is a highly orchestrated response to a perceived threat or challenge that includes biological, behavioral, cognitive, and emotional elements. A stressor is the real or imagined thing that sets off this whole process. Humans are unique in that we can make ourselves incredibly stressed about something that never happened and may never happen.

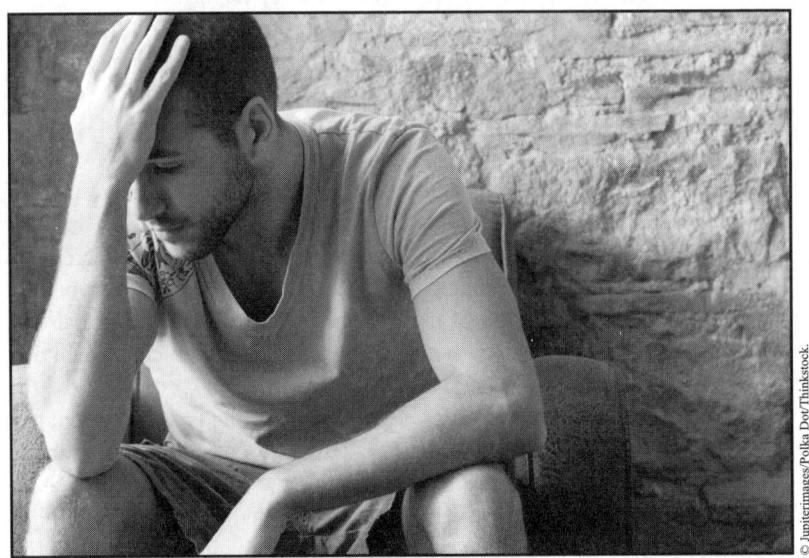

Depression is a disorder that is clearly related to stress.

- There are two complementary biological pathways that mediate the stress response: the sympathetic nervous system and the HPA axis. More specifically, the pathway for the sympathetic nervous system is a sympathoadrenal medullary system (SAM). The sympathetic nervous system activates the adrenal glands—or, specifically, the adrenal medulla—to release epinephrine and norepinephrine, leading to a stress response.

- The best and clearest example of a disease that is related to overarousal of the sympathetic nervous system and, of course, to stress is cardiovascular disease. Other diseases that are clearly related to stress are diabetes, metabolic syndrome, obesity, dyslipidemia, and stress-related disorders such as depression, anxiety, and posttraumatic stress.

The Parasympathetic Nervous System
- Instead of fight or flight, the parasympathetic nervous system is about rest and digest. Its neurotransmitter, or chemical messenger, is acetylcholine—not norepinephrine or epinephrine.

- The parasympathetic nervous system can be stimulated by anything that helps us to relax, including massage, relaxing music, and even hugs from a significant other.

- In 1976, Herb Benson coined the term "relaxation response," which is a decrease in respiration; decrease in heart rate; decrease in blood pressure; decrease in blood to the muscles; and decrease in blood sugar, cortisol, and catecholamines. Essentially, it involves a rationing down of all of these factors, many of which are related to sympathetic nervous system activity and to cardiovascular reactivity.

- For the most part, parasympathetic nervous system activity is measured just by measuring Benson's factors. Those are important, but there's an interesting, relatively new way to try to measure parasympathetic tone with something called heart rate variability, which involves putting a heart monitor on an individual, usually for at least 24 hours, and monitoring their heartbeats.

Suggested Reading

Benson and Klipper, *The Relaxation Response.*

Blessing and Gibbons, "Autonomic Nervous System."

Johnson, *Mind Wide Open.*

Questions to Consider

1. Is the "tend and befriend" response biologically or socially created? How might the world be different if it were equally present in both men and women?

2. Is it possible to permanently lower the set point for sympathetic arousal in an anxious person? If not, how can the person compensate?

Simmering Soup—The Neuroendocrine System
Lecture 4

In this lecture, you're going to learn about the neuroendocrine system, the second half of the stress-response system. The first half involves the autonomic nervous system—in particular, the sympathetic nervous system and its fight-or-flight response. This lecture provides an overview of the endocrine system, which secretes its chemical messengers and hormones into the bloodstream (not outside the body, such as sweat glands or tear ducts). You will learn how the hypothalamic-pituitary-adrenal axis is related to disease and even health.

Endocrine Anatomy: Form

- The hypothalamus sits in that middle level in the mammalian brain, approximately at the center, just above the pituitary gland. The hypothalamus is divided into a number of different sections that are responsible for essential life functions, such as the regulation of temperature, hunger, and thirst; the sleep-wake cycle; the sexual drive; and the stress-response system. The hypothalamus tends to be the first in a cascade or chain of activating events that eventually activates the target organ, such as the adrenal glands to secrete cortisol.

- The pituitary sits just below the hypothalamus, in the base of your skull in an area called the Turkish saddle. It's about the size of a small marble. Your hypothalamus and pituitary together secrete approximately 16 different hormones. We're most interested in the stimulation of the adrenals to release cortisol.

- The thyroid and the parathyroid sit in front of your windpipe just below your voice box. The thyroid is responsible for the regulation of metabolism. The parathyroid is four small marble-shaped objects, just behind the thyroid, that is responsible mostly for the regulation of calcium in the body and are related to things like osteoporosis.

- The adrenals sit on top of your kidneys. They're approximately two inches in length, but there's actually two parts to the adrenals: the adrenal cortex and the adrenal medulla. The medulla is essentially the inside, and that's where the norepinephrine and epinephrine come from. The cortex is the outside, and that's where cortisol, aldosterone, a small amount of sex hormones, and even a little bit of epinephrine and norepinephrine are secreted.

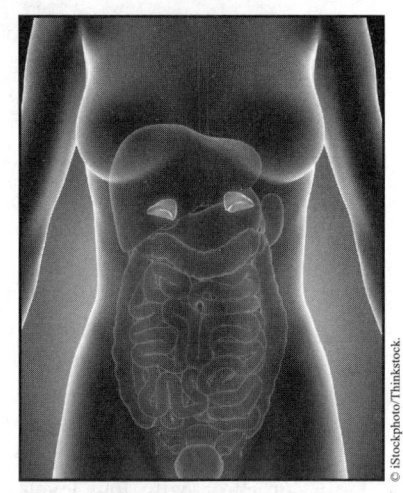

The adrenal glands are responsible for releasing cortisol, which is a stress hormone.

- The pancreas is in your abdomen just behind your stomach. It can be both an exocrine organ as well as an endocrine organ. Endocrine secretes into the blood; exocrine in this sense isn't outside the body, but it's secreting enzymes into the gut. It's responsible for both the secretion of insulin, which pulls down our blood sugar, and glucagon, which can increase our blood sugar.

- The gonads—testes in men and ovaries in women—are responsible for things like estrogen and testosterone. They affect behavior and are most important in terms of reproduction and sex drive. The gonads aren't responsible for turning up or turning down the stress response, but things like libido and reproduction are affected by stress.

Endocrine Anatomy: Function
- Hormones are released into the blood. They can be circulated throughout the body until they reach the target organ or the area of the body that has receptors specifically designed to be stimulated by that hormone.

- Neurotransmitters are primarily how neurons talk to one another over very short distances, from one axon to a dendrite. They're not circulated throughout the body.

- In comparison to neurotransmitters, hormones have a slower onset, have more versatile effects, and can be much longer lasting. They are often the final product in a cascade of messengers.

- We have about 50 different hormones in the body, and each has multiple subtypes of receptors. They can be excitatory or inhibitory, but the picture is much more complex than that.

- It's not just about regulating the level of hormones that may be circulating through our bodies. If we have chronically high or chronically low levels of a hormone, our body responds by producing more or less receptors, so it's either easier or more difficult for that organ to be stimulated.

- The other important part is that we don't want to turn the system on and leave it on. There needs to be some sort of mechanism to turn it back down. In this case, there are a few different feedback loops.

- The first has to do with cortisol receptors. The adrenals will release cortisol, which does its work in the body but also circulates back to the brain—specifically to the hypothalamus. When the hypothalamus is stimulated by cortisol, it realizes that its work has been done. It can now shut down that cascade of events. There's a negative feedback loop.

- The second system is a direct neural connection between the adrenals and the hypothalamus to tell it, again, that its work has been done—that cortisol has been successfully released. Things can now be pulled back down to baseline.

- This bidirectional relationship is not just about turning on or turning off. It's not just about how hormones affect the body. It's also about how those hormones in the body affect the brain.

Hans Selye and HPA Physiology

- In the mid-1920s, Hans Selye was interested in sex hormones and, in particular, how sex hormones affect behavior and development. He primarily used a rodent model. He studied rats to research sex hormones and development.

- Fortunately—for the field, but unfortunately for his lab rats—he was not very good at finding injection sites on his rats or at giving them the appropriate amount of an injection.

- At the end of his experiment, he had a group of incredibly stressed-out rats. He was intrigued by the fact that all of his rats had an enlarged adrenal cortex and that their thymus and lymph nodes seemed to have shrunk. Many of them had ulcers and were more susceptible to developing different types of cancer.

- He eventually called this the general adaptation syndrome, but we know that these are all stress-related diseases. His further research in his career helped us to understand the different stages of the general adaptation syndrome. The first stage is an initial alarm from the sympathetic-adrenal medullary system as well as the hypothalamic-pituitary-adrenal axis (HPA) axis. The second stage is resistance—fight or adaptation, perhaps. After all of your energy has been spent, the third stage, the exhaustion stage, e is when we see some of the chronic diseases that Selye saw in his lab rats.

- We know about HPA physiology because of Selye and his rats. The HPA axis tells us what the pathway is: The hypothalamus releases corticotropin-releasing hormone (CRH) and stimulates the pituitary, which releases adrenocorticotropic hormone (ACTH), which stimulates the adrenals. Eventually, cortisol, which is the stress hormone, is released.

- Cortisol is the second half of the stress-response system. As a hormone, it is much slower to turn on and takes much longer to turn off. It doesn't work in opposition to the sympathetic nervous system; it's seen as a complement to the sympathetic nervous system.

- Many people call cortisol the "Goldilocks hormone" because you have to have just the right amount in order to be healthy. If you have too much, you have health problems; if you have too little, you have health problems.

- Cortisol, much like epinephrine and norepinephrine, has an important impact on cardiovascular function, including an impact on blood pressure—but the effects are slightly different. When cortisol is released, it doesn't directly cause arterial dilation or vasoconstriction. Instead, it makes the endothelium, the lining of the inside of the blood vessels, more sensitive to epinephrine and norepinephrine.

- Despite its effects on the cardiovascular system, cortisol's primary function is in the metabolism or use of carbohydrates, protein, and lipids (fats). Essentially, when an individual has a release of cortisol, they're going to need some energy to fight or flee whatever might be ahead of them.

- First, cortisol causes muscle fibers to be broken down into their constituent amino acids, or building blocks, which are pushed into the bloodstream. They are picked up by the liver, which uses these amino acids to make more glucose in a process called gluconeogenesis. When that glucose is created, it's released into the bloodstream. For the most part, our brain consumes the vast majority of our glucose for energy.

- The second thing that cortisol does is it causes lipids to be released into the bloodstream. If you have preexisting atherosclerosis or high blood pressure, you don't want a cortisol system constantly putting more lipids into your bloodstream. You're worried about blood clots, plaques, and further promotion of atherosclerosis—particularly under situations in which you're chronically stressed and your cortisol is chronically high.

- The last and maybe most important thing that cortisol does is it has an effect on the immune system. Essentially, cortisol is meant to suppress certain aspects of the immune system—specifically inflammation.

Bruce McEwen and Allostasis

- An idea called allostasis, which originated from Bruce McEwen, challenges Walter Cannon's idea of homeostasis. Allostasis is the ability to achieve stability through change. Essentially, it says that if we want to keep things on an even keel, our autonomic nervous system, neuroendocrine system, HPA axis, and immune system always have to be changing.

- Unfortunately, all of this changing creates wear and tear over time, or a measure called allostatic load. We all have allostatic load, and it increases over time as we get older.

- Allostasis is not just about having an amount of a particular neurotransmitter or hormone that is too high or too low. It's also about your level of reactivity. The trigger that activates the stress response can be either too sensitive or insensitive.

- An example of exaggerated reactivity might be someone who is easily angered. An example of inadequate reactivity might be someone who is depressed. It's not just about magnitude or the sensitivity of the trigger; it's also about the duration. You might turn on the stress response, but it lasts for a very long time because you are someone who chronically ruminates and worries.

Suggested Reading

Johnson, *Mind Wide Open.*

McEwen, "Stress, Adaptation, and Disease."

Questions to Consider

1. Is there a way to reverse the cumulative, stress-related wear and tear on the body (i.e., allostatic load)? What interventions might be promising?

2. Are over-the-counter cortisol blockers effective in managing stress or obesity? Why do or why don't they work?

Deploying the Troops—Basic Immunology
Lecture 5

In this lecture, you will learn about the immune system. Just as with previous lectures, you will learn about both anatomy and physiology. You will learn about the form and function of the different players in the immune system. Then, you will learn about how the brain—or, more specifically, the mind—interacts with the immune system, and vice versa. Throughout the lecture, you will learn about infection, inflammation, and wound healing.

The Immune System: Form

- The immune system essentially has three key elements. First, the immune system's purpose is to destroy and clear any foreign organisms, including microbes, infected cells, viruses, and bacteria. Its second purpose is to remove dead and injured tissue, an important part of wound healing. The third purpose is to destroy altered cells in the case of cancer cells or damaged cells.

- The immune system has to accomplish all three of these purposes while carefully discriminating normal self from nonself, and sometimes this doesn't quite work.

- In order to have an effective immune system, we need to have just the right amount of a response. An immune deficit results in increased susceptibility to infection and to cancer. An overactive immune response can result in autoimmune diseases like rheumatoid arthritis, or it can result or contribute to diseases like cardiovascular disease.

- We don't always want to turn up the immune system. Sometimes we want to turn it down, and that's why we have immunosuppressive drugs. In fact, they can be lifesaving in a few different circumstances, including for patients of organ transplants and those with autoimmune diseases, such as lupus.

- As part of the immune system, the tonsils are important for the production as well as the storage of particular immune cells. Even though you can do perfectly well without your tonsils, if you have them removed, you're pulling away some of the potential of the immune system.

- Another part of the immune system is lymph nodes. We have a lot of lymph nodes distributed throughout the body, and they are primarily reservoirs for different immune cells.

- The bone marrow is another important part of our immune system. This is the origin of our white blood cells, or lymphocytes, which are released into our bloodstream on their mission to search and destroy any invader.

- The thymus is where our T cells are differentiated into functioning cells.

- Our spleen is essentially a filtering system for our blood. It helps to produces immune cells. It also helps to store those immune cells to be released whenever they are needed.

- A pathogen is an invader—a virus, bacteria, or fungi—that's going to cause you to have a disease of some sort.

- Lymphocytes are a kind of white blood cell. The large lymphocytes are known as natural killer cells, a nonspecific form of immunity. The small lymphocytes are known as B cells and T cells. These are the slower, more specific immune cells that are a part of our backline immune response.

- The term "antigen" is short for "antibody generator." This isn't a full-blown pathogen; rather, it is a molecule that triggers an immune response and, specifically, an antibody response.

- Antibodies are molecules that react with a specific antigen to either kill or neutralize it.

The Immune System: Function

- The various parts of the immune system work in conjunction with one another to protect us from injury or illness. It's actually a very complex, multilayered response that has both frontline and backline immunity.

- Our first line of defense is our most efficient, but it's one that we often take for granted. Our skin is actually our most effective immune organ. Our skin is essentially a protective coating that keeps pathogens from getting inside our skin. Of course, there are times when you can be injured and have an opening, and we also have openings in our body, so pathogens can find a way to invade.

- If a pathogen does invade, it will immediately encounter our frontline defenses: free, circulating immune cells, primarily called phagocytes and monocytes, whose job is to identify anything that's not you and kill it. Essentially, they will engulf the invader to kill it. Next, they will take an antigen—a piece of the invader—to the backline immune system. Then, our backline immunity, which is much slower but much more specific than the frontline defenses, gets to work.

- Another important process is inflammation, which essentially helps us quarantine an infection site or an injury. Inflammation is a complex set of events that brings immune cells into a damaged area so that they can destroy or inactivate foreign organisms and set the stage for tissue repair.

- The frontline immune organs are the phagocytes and macrophages. The macrophages release a chemical messenger called cytokines, of which there are a number of different subtypes. Cytokines are essentially recruiters or traffic signals that pull more immune cells to that site.

- To get the immune cells to a site of injury, the blood flow to the capillaries around the injury has to increase, and the permeability of those capillaries also increases. The fluid inside the blood and those immune cells actually pass through the lining of the tissues of the capillaries into wherever the injury is. As a result, the area looks swollen and red, and it might be painful.

- There are four characteristics of inflammation: pain (dolor), swelling (tumor), heat (calor), and redness (rubor). Inflammation recruits immune cells and gets them to the site where you've been injured so that they can do their work. They produce dead pathogens, or immune cells, and lots of fluid that we call pus that often needs to be removed from the injury site.

Assessing Immune Function
- There are a number of different ways to assess immune function. One way is to simply count the number of specific cells—T cells, B cells, and macrophages. You might look at an injury site and look at how many of those cells are recruited to that specific injury site, rather than just counting the general number of cells that are freely circulating throughout the body.

- Instead of a number, you might be interested in function. It doesn't matter if you have a lot of immune cells if they're just sitting around and not doing very much. For functioning, you want to know about activation (do they get turned on?), proliferation (are they growing and multiplying?), and cytotoxicity (how effective are they at digesting those different pathogens?).

- Another possibility for measurement is looking at the production of antibodies. There are a few different ways you can use antibodies to measure immune function. The first is by looking at the presence of antibodies to latent viruses. When you measure antibodies for a latent virus and you have higher levels, it means that your immune system is not working as well as it should.

- You can also measure antibodies to a recent vaccination or flu shot, for example. The way most vaccinations and flu shots work is they give you an attenuated, or damaged, virus. It's injected into your body so that it stimulates your backline immune system to start

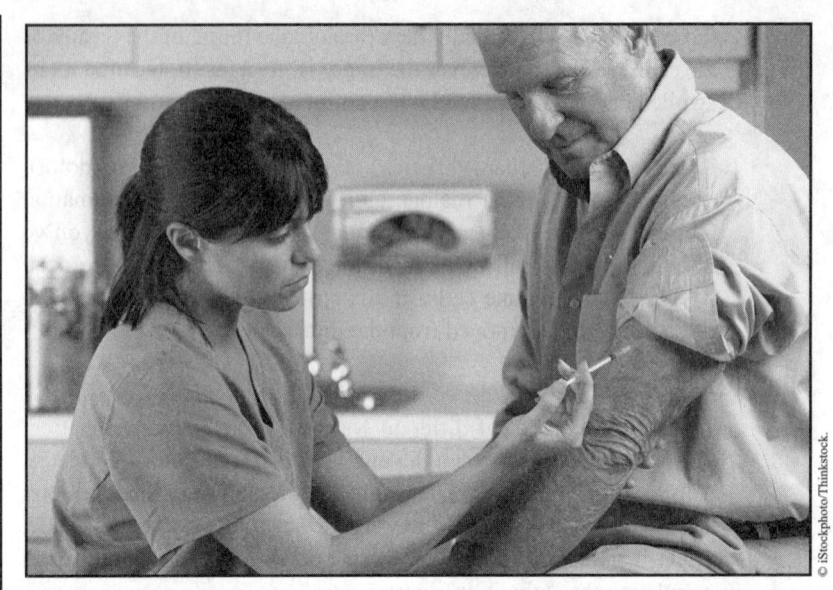

A flu shot contains a damaged version of the virus it is supposed to protect you against.

creating antibodies. If you have a robust immune response, meaning that it creates lots of antibodies, it means that your immune system is working well. After a flu shot, it's a good thing if you see lots of antibodies.

- You can also assess immune function by looking at the products of immune cells, such as the chemical messengers known as cytokines. You can also use direct, more clinical measures. You can look at how often a person catches a cold or how long the flu lasts for a particular individual, for example.

The Immune System and the Mind
- There are a number of different pathways or channels of communication between the mind and the immune system. One of those ways has to do with the receptors that are on the immune cells themselves.

- Immune cells express receptors for products of the HPA axis. Specifically, they can be stimulated or inactivated by cortisol because they have receptors on the actual immune cells themselves. Cortisol also influences immune cell numbers, so it affects proliferation. It also influences immune cell function. In general, certain kinds of immunity are decreased while certain kinds of immunity are increased.

- It's not just about the HPA axis, though. The other half of the stress-response system is the autonomic nervous system. We're looking specifically at the sympathetic nervous system—that fight, flight, or freeze response. Immune cells have receptors for epinephrine and norepinephrine on the actual cells themselves.

- Moreover, nerve fibers from the autonomic nervous system directly innervate immune organs. Your thymus, spleen, and lymph nodes can be directly activated by your autonomic nervous system.

- With the stress-response system and its relationship to the immune function, we have a double-edged sword. If you have too much of the stress hormone cortisol, for example, it can suppress the immune system, and you're going to have an increased incidence of infection and maybe other problems. If you have too little cortisol reactivity, it can impair the ability of the system to constrain inflammation.

Suggested Reading

Abbas, Lichtman, and Pillai, *Basic Immunology*.

Marucha, Kiecolt-Glaser, and Favagehi, "Mucosal Wound Healing Is Impaired by Examination Stress."

Questions to Consider

1. If psychological stress suppresses the immune system, is stress beneficial for people with autoimmune disorders (i.e., overactive immune systems)

or for people who have had organ transplants (i.e., reduces the risk of your body rejecting the organ)?

2. If social support, altruism, and intimacy are all beneficial for our health, why can caregiving be a chronic stressor that harms our health?

Nature vs. Nurture—Genes, Health, and Disease
Lecture 6

In this lecture, you will learn about genetics and, specifically, about a new area of genetic research called epigenetics. The lecture begins with a review of basic genetics and inheritance. Then, you will be introduced to a new behavior-genes pathway, where it's not just that genetics affects our behavior, but it's also that our behavior potentially alters our genetics. You will also be exposed to an exciting new area of epigenetics that involves the possibility of overriding our genetic programming in both terrific and terrible ways.

Basic Genetics

- Gregor Mendel, who studied pea plants, gave us the ideas of genotype and phenotype—of recessive and dominant genes. He gave us the idea of how to draw a family pedigree, where we can predict the physical characteristics, or phenotypes, of the offspring given who the parents were.

- Deoxyribonucleic acid (DNA) serves as the blueprint for life; it gives us instructions on how to build proteins. Our genome is composed of 46 chromosomes, half of which come from our mother and half of which come from our father. All of these chromosomes reside in the nucleus of each cell.

- Chromosomes are made up of proteins in DNA, which is made up of just four nucleotide base pairs—A, C, T, and G—that are composed together in different orders to form a sort of ladder. Each end of that ladder is twisted to give us the classic double-helix shape. There's approximately 10 feet of DNA tightly wound in the nucleus of each and every cell. A gene is simply a section of DNA that codes for a particular protein.

- Genes code for proteins, which are molecules made up of chains of amino acids. There are about 20 types of amino acids. The shape of the protein depends on which acids are connected and in what particular order. There can actually be thousands of different permutations and all sorts of different proteins. Essentially, for a protein, the shape of the protein equals the destiny and the function of the protein.

- The building blocks of life are made up of proteins. Receptors are made of proteins, and they have to be exactly the right shape if they are to be stimulated by their target chemical messenger. The chemical messengers themselves, hormones and neurotransmitters, are also made up of proteins. In addition, enzymes are made up of proteins.

- Evolution is the idea that incremental, step-by-step changes are brought about through a process of natural selection. On his trip to the Galapagos Islands, Charles Darwin discovered that the shape and size of the beaks of different finches are different depending on the source of food that happened to be available on that island.

- Depending on those external characteristics, animals that have a characteristic that helps them survive—that helps them procreate— are more likely to have more offspring. Their genes are more likely to be passed on to the next generation. Over time, we see those incremental changes in the phenotype of the animal.

- For evolution, at least from a classic sense, it's all about mutations— it's all about changes in the sequences of DNA. It's about insertion mutations, deletion mutations, or point mutations. What we've learned recently, though, is that it's much more complicated and much more interesting than that.

- The most informative way to study genetics is through animal studies. The most commonly used nonhumans that are included in genetic studies are fruit flies or different types of roundworms. The reason these are so important and so informative, from a basic science perspective, is we can actually manipulate the genome.

We can cause those mutations to occur. We can look at those basic biological processes that help us to understand gene expression.

- There are a few ways to study, for example, the heritability of different diseases. The most basic way is to construct a family pedigree, much like Gregor Mendel. We can look at the genotypes and phenotypes of the parents and see which of those characteristics are passed on to their offspring.

- A higher level of study is twin studies, which are considered the gold standard of heritability research. There are two types of twins: monozygotic (identical) twins and dizygotic (nonidentical) twins. Monozygotic twins are essentially clones of one another, so they have exactly the same genetic material. Dizygotic twins come from two separate eggs. Essentially, they have the same environment, but they're no more similar than any two siblings would be.

Epigenetics and Behavioral Genetics

- Histones are a type of protein. You can think of a histone as a spool, and you wrap the DNA, the thread, around that particular spool. Remember that there are 10 feet of DNA in the nucleus of each cell, so things have to be wrapped fairly tightly.

- Chromatin is composed of both chromosomes and proteins. Using the metaphor of spool and thread, we most likely have multiple spools and multiple threads. They all have to be fitted together somehow in that sewing kit—inside the nucleus of the cell. The chromatin's shape can be changed; the architecture can be restructured. If you think about that sewing kit, if you move certain spools to the front or to the back, they're going to be more or less accessible.

- DNA tags can essentially be thought of as "on" or "off" switches, where something new, usually a methyl group, is attached to a piece of DNA. Attaching something new to that piece of thread is going to influence whether or not it can be wound off of that spool and opened up for transcription. If you can't get to the thread and open it up, then you can't make the proteins and the gene is not expressed.

- In epigenetics, the regulation of genome activity is independent of sequence manipulation. We're not moving around those base pairs; we're not cutting, splicing, and inserting.

- Epigenetics is critical in developmental biology. We're born with a lot of genes that are never expressed—that we don't use at all. In the past, we referred to this as "junk DNA," but we actually found out that these genes just haven't been turned on yet. It depends on DNA tags and whether those switches have been turned on or off.

- Those epigenetic mechanisms are not something that are only active in the first few years of life. Epigenetic mechanisms can be active throughout our entire life span. Moreover, once those modifications are affixed to your genetic material, they can be passed on transgenerationally.

- If you and your partner have offspring, you're going to pass on your genetic material to your child. You might not think, though, about how your life choices—how your behaviors—might have altered your genetic material within your lifetime and that those alterations are going to be inherited by your children.

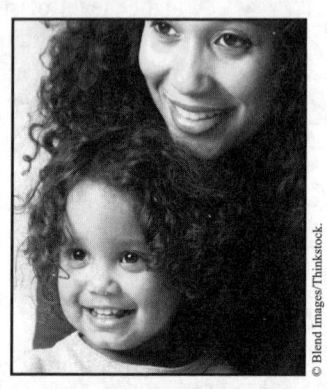

During pregnancy, the health of the mother matters, so prenatal care is important.

- There are a few different mechanisms of epigenetics. The first mechanism has to do with DNA tags, which are also called epigenetic marks. With this mechanism, we're not focused on changes in the DNA sequence; we're focused on changes in the DNA molecule itself and the structures that determine accessibility of DNA to transcription.

- The second mechanism for epigenetics is called histone modification, which influences how tightly the DNA can be wrapped around the spool, with loose wrapping potentially making genes more open and available to transcription.

- Behavioral genetics is a very fascinating study of how genetics influences our behavior. Epigenetics has shown us that there is a bidirectional pathway between genes and behavior: Genes influence behavior, but behavior can also influence genetic expression.

Gene-Environment Interaction

- The idea of transgenerational inheritance refers to the ability of environmental factors to promote a phenotype, or physical characteristics, in subsequent progeny and successive generations. The chemical tags—the methylation of cytosine on a DNA molecule, the modification of histones, and the acetylation or methylation of those histones—are captured within the DNA of the eggs and sperm, and they can be conveyed to the next generation.

- If we have healthy behaviors, such as exercising and eating well, it's possible that these behaviors could be passed on to our offspring. Unfortunately, this can also happen in the opposite direction. If we have unhealthy behaviors, or even if we've suffered a severe trauma in our lifetime that has caused epigenetic modifications to our DNA, it's possible that those modifications then can be passed on to subsequent generations.

- Another area of research is called fetal origins research, which involves studying how the in utero environment affects the adult individual. We know that the health of the mother matters because the fetus is particularly vulnerable during this period of very rapid development. However, it goes much further than that.

- There is a new area of research in the realm of gene-environment interaction called telomere research. A telomere is a region of repetitive nucleotide sequences at each end of a chromosome that protects the chromosome from deterioration. Research has shown that there are a number of outside stressors that affect telomere length. There may be ways to slow down telomere shortening and possibly take away some of the physical consequences of stress.

- In modern times, there is a lot of talk about genomic medicine and gene therapies. The idea of personalized medicine is that as it becomes easier and cheaper to map the entire genome of an individual, we should have the opportunity for early identification of genetic risk for different sorts of diseases. This can be very helpful, but it can also cause a great deal of stress and anxiety.

Suggested Reading

Paul, *Origins*.

Tollefsbol, *Epigenetics in Human Disease*.

Questions to Consider

1. Under what conditions should genetic screening for disease risk be declined? Would you want to know your full genetic disease risk profile?

2. Could epigenetic therapies be developed to treat or prevent disease? What are some of the ethical and practical concerns?

Forget Me Not—Cognitive Function
Lecture 7

The focus of this lecture is cognition and intellectual functioning. This lecture will define the construct of IQ and teach you about how it can be measured and whether it is changeable. You will also learn some potential exercises—both cognitive exercises as well as physical exercises—that might actually improve and change cognitive functioning. Finally, you will learn about memory and learning: Neurons that fire together wire together; this is how we learn.

Intelligence and IQ

- In general, intelligence refers to intellectual functioning, which includes memory, creativity, problem solving, abstract thought, reasoning, and so on. It includes the skills of attention, concentration, information processing, conceptualizing a problem, and novel thinking.

- Some percentage of intelligence, or maybe the intelligence quotient (IQ), is rooted in our biology—our genetic inheritance. Our intellectual functioning resides in our brain and specifically in our minds, both of which are highly influenced by our environment.

- Raymond Cattell was a psychologist who was very interested in intellectual functioning and intelligence. He talked about a general intelligence factor, or *g* factor. This served as the precursor for our modern notion of IQ. He believed that a *g* factor included both fluid intelligence and crystalline intelligence.

- Fluid intelligence is about fluid, flexible problem solving. It's about being able to think logically and cleverly about new math problems that you maybe haven't seen before. The second form of intelligence, crystalline intelligence, is about accumulated experience, or knowledge. This is probably where wisdom resides—learning how to apply the knowledge that we've gained.

In general, fluid intelligence decreases with age while crystalline intelligence increases with age.

- IQ is a measure of intellectual functioning. The first mass IQ testing was in 1917, and it was done to screen potential soldiers being recruited or drafted to World War I. They needed a quick-and-easy way to separate the potential recruits who should go on to be officers and those who should be privates. This was the Stanford-Binet Intelligence Scale, which was created by Lewis Terman.

- Another intelligence test is the Wechsler Adult Intelligence Scale (WAIS). Both the Stanford-Binet and the WAIS are divided into a number of different subscales that help illuminate people's cognitive strengths and weaknesses.

- For the most part, IQ tests are based on an average score of 100 with a standard deviation of 15. This means that you're still considered in the normal IQ range if you have an IQ of between 85 and 115. You are considered a "genius" if you have an IQ of 130 or higher. However, it's important to remember that there are plenty of average people who are doing some incredible things.

- IQ scores have been associated with a number of different factors, including morbidity and mortality. As your IQ score goes up, your risk for morbidity and mortality goes down.

- IQ scores are also related to parental IQ and social status. IQ scores, although not the main determinant of academic performance, account for about 25 percent of the variance.

- When you look at success in general, IQ has an even lower correlation. When you look at things like having successful relationships or having a high quality of life, there's essentially no relationship between IQ and those variables.

- Education can actually boost IQ somewhat. By enrolling low-income children in a head-start program, their IQs can jump by as

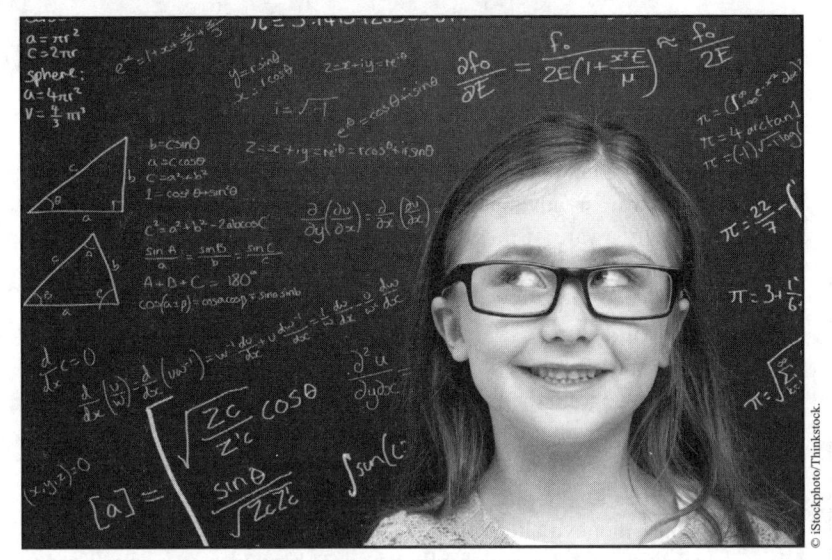

Can IQ be accurately measured? Is it changeable?

much as 13 points. In addition, education can help you keep your intelligence longer. In essence, you use it or you lose it. If you want to keep your IQ up, you have to keep learning.

- Genetics also plays an important part with IQ. To date, we don't have great epigenetic studies that examine the relationship between epigenetics and IQ, but stay tuned.

- There are some fascinating studies coming out of the University of California, Davis, that look at antioxidants as well as omega-3 fatty acids and cognitive functioning. It looks like there might be an important link.

- On the other hand, if you're exposed to neurotoxins during critical periods of development—for example, in a prenatal environment, in your infancy, or in childhood—it could have a damaging effect on your IQ.

- In addition, socioeconomic status and, particularly, poverty can have a very depressive effect on IQ, but we can reverse it.

- Of course, these factors don't occur in isolation. Often, many of them are happening at the same time. Sometimes these social pressures, or advantages, happen behind the scenes, and we're not fully aware of them, even though they may be lifting us up or pushing us down.

Training the Mind
- There are a number of factors that influence intellectual functioning, but can we train the mind? The short answer to that is yes.

- Neurobics is aerobics for your neurological system—to improve cognitive functioning. There is a new category of software that's a big moneymaker called brain-training software. With this software, they have basically taken the structure of an intelligence test and broken it down into different kinds of intellectual skills or functioning, such as vocabulary tests and 3-D image rotation.

- Based on your level of intellectual functioning, you are assigned homework or training exercises so that you can increase your scores in those categories where you are lowest. You're also given the opportunity to practice in those categories where you were strongest to stay strong in those areas.

- In addition to brain-training software, there are many ways that you can go about training your mind and increasing or improving your cognitive functioning. One example is learning a new language. Another example is learning to play a musical instrument, particularly if you've never played a musical instrument before. You also might do crossword puzzles or sudoku.

- The effect sizes are small, but in randomized controlled trials, we see that cognitive function actually does increase from these relatively simple interventions. The effect sizes might be small, but the effects are long lasting—and hopefully you have fun along the way.

- Physical exercise has a medium effect size. It doesn't have to be a fancy program; you don't need any sort of neurocognitive assessment of your intellectual functioning. What you need to do is primarily aerobic exercise.

- The benefits of exercise, in terms of improved intellectual functioning, tend to decline when the exercise ends—unlike neurobics.

- Exercise also decreases the risk for dementia, which is defined as changes in intellectual functioning with age—specifically, declines with age. One in eight adults over the age of 65 have some signs of dementia, with Alzheimer's disease being the most common. Interventions like diet, exercise, neurobics, stress reduction, social activities, community engagement, and other exercises work—not as a cure, but at least in terms of slowing things down.

Memory and Learning
- We have both short-term and long-term memory. There are many strategies that help us improve our short-term memory, including rehearsal. If someone tells you his or her phone number, the way to remember it is just to repeat it over and over again.

- Long-term memory is a little more complex. Long-term memory is the keyboard to the computer that enters in new memories. Emotions influence whether or not we learn memories and how memory traces are laid down. When we recall memories, it's also about our emotional state at the time—it's not just about facts. Memories are very much fallible.

- We have explicit memories, also called declarative memories, which are about factual or semantic information. We have implicit memories, which might be about emotions, subtle social perceptions, priming, procedural skills, or motor memory (such as learning to play the piano).

- In all of these cases of memory, neurons that fire together wire together. It's all about neuroplasticity, which refers to changes in neural architecture—an increase or decrease in the number of neurons, their interconnections, and changes in their patterns of firing.

- Learning is more than just remembering facts. In fact, there's a phenomenon in medical school called intellectual bulimia, where students binge on tons of facts right before a test and memorize them for the short term. They purge on the test, and then they promptly forget half of what they learned.

- What about the biopsychosocial model in memory and learning? The biological pathways—the sympathetic nervous system (fight or flight), the HPA axis and stress, the hippocampus and cortisol—all influence our capacity for memory or learning.

Suggested Reading

Breedlove, Watson, and Rosenzsweig, *Biological Psychology*.

Duncan, *How Intelligence Happens*.

Hurley, "Can You Make Yourself Smarter?"

Questions to Consider

1. What are the potential positive and negative implications of attaching an IQ score to a particular child? Is there a better alternative to assess intellectual functioning?

2. Are we currently experiencing a sharp rise in the prevalence of Alzheimer's disease and other forms of dementia, or are we just looking for it more carefully now? If there has been a rise in the prevalence, then why?

Mind over Matter—Cognition in Everyday Life
Lecture 8

In this lecture, you will learn about one of the products of intellectual functioning: cognition. You will learn about different types of cognition, and you will be exposed to some examples of cognition. You will focus on specific kinds of cognition, such as the placebo effect and the power of belief, and how these types of cognitions can affect your health. You will also learn about cognitive processing—specifically, the dual-process model of thinking, which involves system-one and system-two thinking. You will also examine cognitive behavioral therapy.

Cognition and Cognitive Processes

- Cognition includes any activity of the mind. It can be words, images, sounds, attitudes or beliefs, generalizations, stereotypes, scripts or schemas, expectations, attributions, or appraisals. It can be intuition, assumptions, or even automatic thoughts.

- At times, placebos can have very profound effects on our health—but is the placebo about expectation or perception? Is it something that's simply imaginary? The classic placebo studies are about pain and the experience of pain, usually acute pain.

- For example, you recruit a group of subjects that have lower back pain. You give all of the subjects a bottle of pills. Half of them are receiving opiates, something like Vicodin, for their back pain. The other half, unbeknownst to them, have received sugar pills.

- You ask both groups how well the pills work, and both of them—the

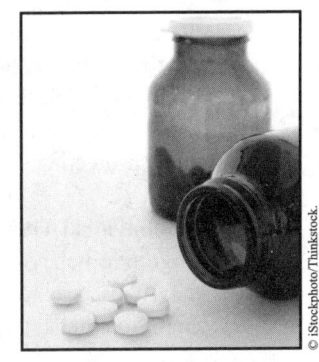

A placebo is a sugar pill that does not contain any medication.

placebo group and the group that received the real drug—will say that their pain has decreased. It's probably about perception, but there also seems to be some sort of biological alteration that's occurring.

- In cognitive psychology, the dual-process model of thinking compares system-one thinking with system-two thinking. System one is very quick, automatic, and intuitive, but we make a lot of snap judgments that might not be correct. System two is much slower and more rational. It's much more accurate, but it takes a lot more time and energy.

- We all have habits of mind. Our system-one thinking is reflexive thinking that sometimes lifts us up and sometimes pushes us down. Some people will overpersonalize things that happen. Sometimes we only selectively attend to information that fits our preexisting beliefs. We may have all-or-none thinking: A person is all good or all bad.

- We try to read other people's minds and imagine what they're thinking—sometimes accurately but often not—and we try to predict the future. These habits of mind are shortcuts. They can make things more efficient, but they can also cause problems.

- From a recent survey, approximately 90 percent of men think they're in the top 50 percent of social skills. In addition, 90 percent of drivers think they're above average. Some have said that maybe these distortions are like having a psychological immune system that's protecting its host from threats to its self-esteem.

Cognitive Behavioral Therapy

- Cognitive behavioral therapy, which has been around since about the 1970s, teaches us to understand the interrelationships between cognition, behavior, and emotions.

- The way people's thoughts affect the way they feel affect the things they do. This interdependence between thoughts, behavior, and emotions is important because if we want to change an emotion, we can change a thought or a behavior—or we can do a little of both.

- Cognitive behavioral therapy stems from the work of Aaron Beck and others, who tell us that humans are imperfect information processors that typically develop nonnormative habits of mind (sometimes called dysfunctional thinking). This is system-one thinking, and it is common—not abnormal. However, if used too often, it can cause psychological difficulty, such as depression and anxiety.

- Many of us operate on a noncognitive model. We will say something like, "John made me so angry"—as if the situation reached into your brain, stimulated your limbic system, and made you angry.

- We know from a cognitive model that there's actually a middle step that happens. There's a situation—John and whatever he did—but then there's the way you interpret it. You have automatic thoughts, which we don't rationally create or generate; instead, they just pop into our mind, almost like a reflex.

- The way you feel is actually a product of the situation and the automatic thought. The reason that this is good news is because those automatic thoughts occur inside us, and we have an opportunity to retrieve them and maybe do something to change them.

- How is cognition related to emotions? If an individual is prone to feeling anxious, he or she probably often misperceives threats that might be in his or her environment. He or she may also underestimate his or her capacity to cope or the resources or social supports that are available.

- For an individual who is depressed, we often see something called the negative cognitive triad. Depression is about, essentially, the perception of a real or symbolic loss. With the negative cognitive triad, we have negative thoughts that tend to occur in three different areas: about the self, about others, and about the world being an unfriendly, hostile, unsupportive place.

- These thoughts are usually measured by questionnaires like the Dysfunctional Attitude Scale (DAS), which is composed of 100 questions on a one to seven scale. A sample question is as follows: "Most people are okay once you get to know them." You rate this on a scale of one to seven whether you agree with that belief.

Learned Helplessness and Attributional Style
- Learned helplessness is a type of cognition that can have profound impacts on an individual's health. However, it is also amenable to cognitive behavioral therapy.

- In the late 1960s and early 1970s, Martin Seligman conducted learned helplessness experiments by looking at dogs. This was the basic experimental paradigm. He would have a large rectangular cage. On one side of the cage, there was a metal floor. On the other side of the cage, there was a nonmetallic floor.

- There was a divider that could be placed, if the researchers wanted, between those two halves of the cage. They would put the dog in the metal side of the cage and administer electric shock. The dog would immediately jump to the other side to escape. The shock was mildly painful, so this was just a reflex. They do this multiple times, and the dog jumps to the other side every time.

- In the next part of the experiment, researchers put the divider in the cage and put the dog on the metal side. They administer the shock. The dog jumps against the divider, but there's no way to escape. They administer the shock again, and the dog jumps against the divider and finds that, again, there's no way to escape. Eventually, the dog gives up. It knows there's no way to escape.

- In the third part of the experiment, and the most dramatic part, researchers pull out the divider. They administer a shock to the dog, and the dog just sits there. The researchers think that perhaps the dog doesn't realize that he can now escape, so they physically drag the dog to the other side of the cage to show him that he can now get away from that shock.

- Then, they put him back on the metal side, administer the shock, and the dog does nothing. The dog has learned to be helpless. He has given up, even though his circumstances have now changed.

- If we are to move this phenomenon to humans, it's not difficult to see how this might work. We've all certainly been in situations that were beyond our control. In cases of childhood abuse or neglect, not all of those children go on to develop learned helplessness. In fact, some of them can be quite resilient.

- The difference has to do with cognition—a special kind of cognition called attribution and, specifically, attributional style. The idea is that we have a habitual way in which we explain why events occur. Those children that think their abuse is their fault and that all children are abused go on to develop learned helplessness. The children that believe that their abuse is not their fault and that things are better elsewhere are resilient.

- The research of Martin Seligman and his group on students with low socioeconomic status shows that early intervention to change attributional style can decrease the risk for behavioral problems, increase academic performance, and decrease the risk for depression.

Positive Psychology
- Positive thinking is certainly not a new notion. The power of positive thought was the hallmark of the work of Norman Vincent Peale. But positive thinking actually goes back much before him. Hippocrates talked about the importance of having a positive attitude. Ben Franklin also talked about it.

- There is scientific data that links positive thinking and health. There are a number of studies that are part of a new field of psychology called positive psychology.

Suggested Reading

Beck, *Cognitive Therapy*.

Greenberger and Padesky, *Mind over Mood*.

Satterfield, *A Cognitive-Behavioral Approach to the Beginning of the End of Life*.

———, *Minding the Body*.

Questions to Consider

1. How is cognitive therapy different from old-time sophistry? Is it just mental gymnastics to fool yourself into feeling better?

2. Are there any benefits to depressive or anxious thinking? When should we ride these thoughts out instead of trying to change them?

Emotions Revealed—Psychology of Emotions
Lecture 9

In this lecture, you are going to learn what defines emotions. You are also going to learn about the psychology of emotions: What are their functions, and how do we assess them? In addition, you will review the connection between emotions, cognitions, and behaviors. You will learn about the function and the universality of emotions as well as the various ways people use emotions to communicate what they are feeling.

What Are Emotions?

- Emotions are sources of information. They're intended to communicate information about relationships to the self and the world. You can think of emotions as a sort of weather report; they give us a status of current affairs and help us prepare for possibly stormy weather to come.

- Emotions are meant to motivate either withdrawal or approach. Feeling love brings you closer to a person while feeling fear pushes you further away.

- Emotions influence learning and memory. They are phylogenetically old, meaning that they have deep evolutionary roots. Emotions emerge developmentally, and they're probably very much hardwired early on. For example, even blind infants make facial expressions that match what they're feeling.

- Emotions are linked with thoughts and behaviors in a triangle. If you want to understand emotions, you need to look at what you're thinking and what you're doing. What is the function or purpose of primary emotions? What is the theme or signal they're sending to us?

- Knowing these themes or meanings may help us use emotional information, but there are a number of other steps that we need to take. First, we need to be able to perceive and correctly identify the emotion. This might include physical, cognitive, or behavioral cues. Secondly, we need to know the trigger for that emotion. Was it coming from inside or outside? Was it real or imagined? Did it take place in the present, or is it something from our memories?

- Once you've identified the emotion and its trigger, you've reached the interpretive step, and understanding those themes or functions associated with emotions might help you understand what's going on. Of course, emotions are complex, and they vary greatly across people. It behooves each of us to develop a deep understanding of our emotional instrument.

Basic Emotions
- In the 1960s, Paul Ekman, a psychologist at the University of California, San Francisco, found that the common element of emotions across all cultures was facial expressions. We use facial expressions to communicate emotions, and of course, we all have the same anatomy.

- Ekman took pictures of his graduate students making a variety of different facial expressions: sadness, happiness, surprise, and fear. He then took this portfolio of pictures and went on a tour around the world, stopping at a number of places where they had different languages, cultures, levels of industrialization.

- Through a translator, he would tell a story that was culturally appropriate. He then asked participants to look through his portfolio of pictures and choose the facial expression that matched the story. Subjects had a very easy time doing that with some of the emotions, but not with some of the other emotions.

- From his experiments, Ekman and his colleagues were able to pull out what he called six primary emotions: happiness, surprise, sadness, anger, disgust, and fear. He makes an analogy to primary colors: Six isn't a whole lot, but we can blend those colors, or emotions, together to create all sorts of different hues and shades.

For example, the blended emotion of contempt is most likely composed of anger and disgust.

- Ekman set out to number all of the facial muscles and actually trained himself to independently move all 50 or so facial muscles. He used his knowledge of facial musculature to create essentially a catalog of the different muscles that are recruited to express each and every emotion genuinely. He then started looking at how that atlas differed if a person was faking an emotion.

Verbal and Nonverbal Communication
- In addition to facial expressions, verbal content is important. What are the actual words that are chosen? What is the volume, tone, pitch, prosody, or musicality?

- We, of course, can read emotions over the phone, when there's no visual stimulus whatsoever. We can even sense emotions in a language other than our own, but, of course, we probably make a lot more misinterpretations.

- Another kind of emotional communication is nonverbal communication. Of course, facial expressions are an example of that, but there's actually more than that.

- In fact, in any sort of social exchange, the majority of information that is exchanged between two individuals is primarily nonverbal. We have facial expressions, but we also have body posture.

- We also have subtle clues or signals that are attached when we are attending to what the other person is saying—such as making eye contact or nodding your head—that encourages the person to continue communicating with us.

Physiologic Signatures of Emotions
- The valence of an emotion is the positivity or negativity of the emotion. If we're thinking about health, the valence of an emotion might be important.

- You can group discrete physiologic signatures of emotions into at least a few families. The first family is the family of negative emotions, including depression, anxiety, fear, anger, jealousy, and envy. The word "negative" refers to potential social consequences as well as the dysphoric, or unpleasant, physical sensation they often create.

- Many of these negative emotions are thought to have an evolutionary advantage for survival. Negative emotions or negative feelings are critically important to the fight-or-flight response, for example.

- There's also a physiologic family of emotions called positive emotions, including happiness, joy, love, and excitement. Again, these have a physiologic impact as well as social consequences. In general, these are pleasant to experience.

- Barbara Fredrickson created the broaden-and-build theory to help us understand the evolutionary function of the positive emotion family. There are two parts to it: the "broaden" part and the "build" part.

- The "broaden" part: When an individual is in a negative emotional state, he or she essentially develops cognitive tunnel vision. When an individual is in a positive emotional state, however, we don't see this super focus on just one thing in our environment; instead, we see an opening of our cognitive repertoire—a broadening of the things that we notice (also making you more creative and better at solving problems).

- The "build" part: When you are in a positive emotional state, you're more open to meeting other people, even if you're introverted. Essentially, positive emotions help us build those social relationships that we might need in the tough times ahead.

- Most of us think of negative and positive emotions on a single continuum: negative at one end and positive at the other. As the negative goes down, the positive goes up, and vice versa. However, that doesn't quite hold true.

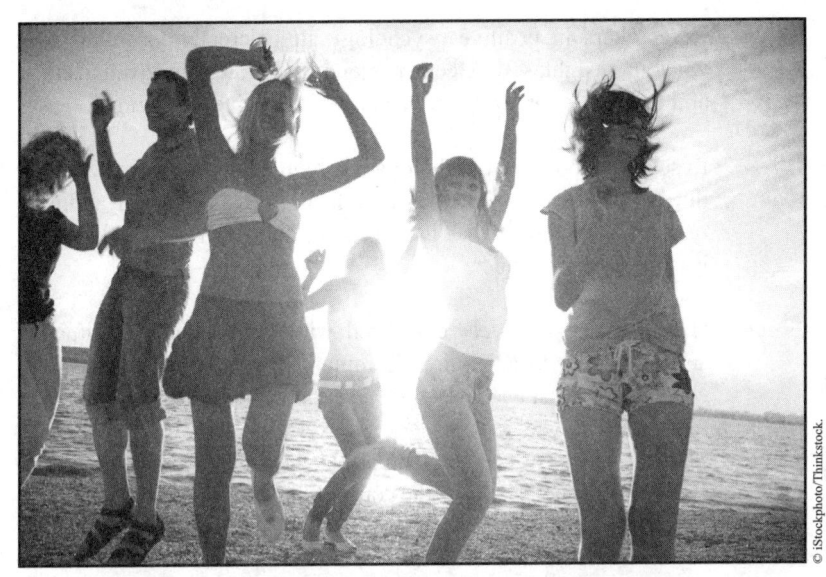

Approximately one-third of Americans would describe themselves as happy.

- When we look at this in experimental settings, or even when we interview people about their emotional states, we find that people can actually have high levels of negative and positive emotions at the same time—maybe not at exactly the same moment. People can have intensely positive and negative things happening in their lives, and they can have feelings about both of those in the same hour, day, or week.

- Preventing a negative emotion doesn't necessarily create a positive emotion; a positive emotion is somehow more than just the absence of a negative emotion. In fact, current emotion researchers are thinking of negative and positive emotions on two separate continua.

Happiness
- The father of positive psychology is Martin Seligman, who brought us the ideas of learned helpfulness and attributional style. This was the guy who was shocking dogs and making them helpless.

- Researchers in positive psychology study creativity, enthusiasm, wisdom, insight, self-esteem, personal and professional satisfaction, and happiness (or, as it's often called, subjective wellbeing).

- Research in positive psychology has found that approximately one-third of Americans would describe themselves as happy. In addition, research has shown that happiness is not generally predicted by income, age, or gender.

- Happiness is positively correlated with extroversion, spirituality, and belonging to a religious community. It is believed that those correlations exist because of social supports and relationships.

- Although age isn't generally correlated with happiness, there do seem to be two peaks over the course of an individual's life in terms of when they're happiest: in your 20s and in your 60s.

- Income and happiness don't seem to be related. If a person has more financial security, then he or she will be a lot happier—up to a certain point. Ultimately, happiness is more than just simple hedonic pleasure. Perhaps it's about things like relationships or meaning, which aren't really tied to income.

Suggested Reading

Ekman, *Emotions Revealed*.

Seligman, *Flourish*.

———, *Learned Optimism*.

Questions to Consider

1. Why is it that negative emotions are "stickier" than positive emotions? Is there anything we could or should do about it?

2. Why do Americans seem so obsessed with being happy? Is this a misguided goal? What goal would be more appropriate?

Agony and Ecstasy—Biology of Emotion
Lecture 10

In this lecture, you will learn about physiologic signatures for emotions. As you will learn in this lecture, emotions may actively alter our memories and how we learn. The link between cognition and emotion is bidirectional. Physiologic arousal is important, but how we explain our emotional arousal is perhaps even more important as we try to explain our experience of emotion and how it affects our health. You are going to learn about a number of different theories that have tried to link the biological with the psychological experience of emotion.

The Biology of Emotions

- Emotions are more than just a feeling. They are a whole-body phenomenon that activates our central nervous system, our limbic system, and even our frontal lobes. They involve neural transmitters and hormones, and they affect the immune system, cardiovascular system, and other bodily systems.

- The biology of emotion resides in both the autonomic nervous system and the central nervous system. Within the autonomic nervous system, the sympathetic nervous system is responsible for the activation of the fight-or-flight response whereas the parasympathetic nervous system pulls us back down.

- Within the central nervous system, the biology of emotions involves the brain—specifically, the limbic system, which includes the amygdala, hippocampus, and thalamus. In addition, this lecture will introduce a new area of the brain called the prefrontal cortex.

- The amygdala is an almond-shaped structure that is responsible for fear and fear-based memories. The hippocampus is the keyboard to the computer that helps us enter in new memories.

- The thalamus is a spherical structure located just above the hippocampus that essentially serves as a sensory relay station. It receives new sensory signals—including visual and auditory signals—copies them, and sends them to different parts of the brain for processing.

- The large lobe in the front of the brain is called the frontal lobe, which is the youngest part of the brain. It's not fully developed until age 25, and it's responsible for executive thinking, or rational thought. The prefrontal cortex is located at the front of the frontal lobes.

- The hippocampus consists of two horns that curve back from the amygdala. It appears to be very important in converting things that are in your mind at the moment (short-term memory) to things that you will remember for a long time (long-term memory). Damage to our hippocampus may prevent us from forming any new memories.

- The hippocampus doesn't really generate emotions, but it's influenced heavily by emotions. If you have chronic levels of stress, it's going to turn down the hippocampus. New research on posttraumatic stress disorder and hippocampal shrinkage suggests that there is a relationship between the two, but we don't know which comes first.

- There is one amygdala in each hemisphere. They are almond-shaped masses of neurons on either side of the thalamus at the lower end of the hippocampus.

- When the amygdala is stimulated electrically, animals respond with aggression. If the amygdala is removed, animals become very tame and can no longer respond to things that would have normally caused rage before. They also lose their adaptive fear response.

- An example of amygdalas in action is flashbulb memories. For example, you may have flashbulb memories from the day that

John F. Kennedy was assassinated. Flashbulb memories are often inaccurate. The amygdala is fairly quick, but it's also fairly messy.

- The prefrontal cortex is the front of the frontal lobe. Brain areas in the region of the prefrontal cortex include the orbital frontal cortex. The prefrontal cortex, and especially the orbital frontal cortex, is very closely connected to our limbic system, and it's a bidirectional relationship.

- The prefrontal cortex appears to play a critical role in the regulation of emotion and behavior by anticipating the consequences of our actions. The prefrontal cortex may also play an important role in delayed gratification by maintaining emotions over time and organizing behavior toward a specific goal.

- There are two hemispheres of the brain, so we have a right and a left prefrontal cortex. If we see increased activation of the right prefrontal cortex, we have more negative emotions, or withdrawal behaviors. The right prefrontal cortex activity is also correlated with more amygdala activity.

- The left prefrontal cortex is associated with more positive emotional states, or the tendency to approach. It is associated with things like meditation and relaxation. Damaging the prefrontal cortex increases an individual's risk for depression.

Emotions in the Body
- The question of whether there's a body signature for each emotion is sort of the holy grail of psychophysiology research. It would be convenient and exciting if we were able to say that anger causes specific muscles to tense, activates particular brain areas, or causes certain changes in biochemistry.

- We haven't found that yet, but there seems to be a negative family and a positive family. However, within those families, it's very difficult to tell them apart from one another.

- Maybe there's a profile of genuine emotions and how they are expressed through musculatures throughout our body. Maybe it has to do with posture. If you think about how your body reshapes itself when you feel an emotion, this point might be clear.

- For example, when you are angry, you make yourself bigger. You stand up straighter, and your shoulders usually go back. Often, the hands are clenched. The chin goes up, and eye contact is usually fairly direct. It's the reverse with embarrassment or shame. Of course, there are facial expressions and facial musculature changes that go with the body changes.

- Other body signatures that we see are changes in body temperature, heart rate, and blood pressure. We also see changes in galvanic skin response, in which the electrical conductance of the outside of your skin changes based on the moisture level of your skin. Although we're often not aware of it, we often are sweating just ever so slightly, and that slight amount of sweat triggered by emotions will change the electrical conductance.

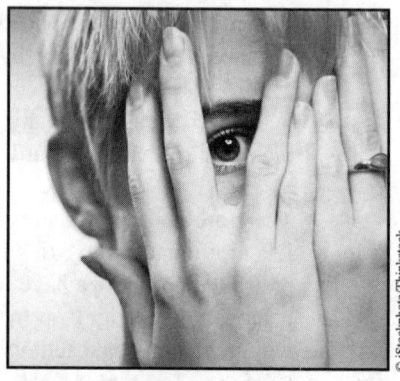

When someone is embarrassed or ashamed, he or she might unconsciously try to hide from view.

Measuring Body Responses

- There are many ways to measure body responses, but there are questions about the validity of some of these tests. Probably the best example is polygraph tests, or lie detectors, which measure heart rate, blood pressure, temperature, and galvanic skin response. The idea is that if an individual is lying, his or her body will tell you so because many of those variables will go off. Even though a person's mind can tell a lie, his or her body cannot.

- Unfortunately, there's actually no good validity data that polygraph tests work at all. Polygraph tests are good for showing when a person is aroused or not aroused. A person could be somewhere in the negative family of emotions, but a polygraph test couldn't tell if the person is lying or telling the truth.

- Biofeedback equipment can measure all sorts of different bodily systems, including galvanic skin response, heart rate, blood pressure, temperature, and muscle tension. Once you're hooked up to the monitors, different psychological strategies can be used to make those variables go down or come up. We learn that we can control our bodily responses.

- Interoception is the perception or the states of your internal organs. This includes if you have any pain in your abdomen or stomach, for example, but also includes things like the sensation of hunger or satiety. Some people are very sensitive to these while others are not. In general, the capacity for interoception decreases with age.

- Proprioception is the perception of your body's position in space. This is something that most people don't often think of. This includes changes in body posture when you're ashamed or angry.

The Biology versus the Psychology of Emotions

- There are three main dueling theories that try to help us understand the relationship between the biology of emotions and the psychology of emotions.

- The first theory, from the late 1800s, is called the James-Lange theory of emotion, which was developed by William James and Carl Lange. It says that the physical expression, or the behavior, actually comes before the emotional or psychological experience. We feel sad because we cry. It still hasn't been clearly proven or disproven.

- The second theory is the Cannon-Bard theory, which takes us back to Walter Cannon and his fight-or-flight response. He believed that emotions originate in the central nervous system, with the resulting emotional experience growing out of unconscious neurological activity. This was based on his work with the rats.

- Both the James-Lange theory and the Cannon-Bard theory focus on the physiology and how the physiology shapes the psychology.

- The Schachter-Singer theory, which was proposed in 1962, is another physiologically based theory of emotion that includes the potentially critical element of cognitive appraisal. In this view, the physiologic arousal associated with emotion was basically generic. The individual perceives the arousal and labels it as a particular emotion based on a cognitive appraisal of the current situation. Physiology is critical to emotion, but the appraisal process is the key.

- For example, you might say that your heart is racing and you're running from an alligator, so therefore, you're afraid. Alternatively, you could say that your heart is racing and you just asked someone out on a date, so you're excited and nervous. It's the same kind of physiologic arousal, but a different appraisal, so you get a different emotional state.

- All of these theories are probably correct to some extent. Emotions are about what happens in both our brain—the limbic system and the prefrontal cortex—and our body.

Suggested Reading

Breedlove, Watson, and Rosenzsweig, *Biological Psychology*.

Damasio, *Looking for Spinoza*.

Ekman, *Emotions Revealed*.

Johnson, *Mind Wide Open*.

Questions to Consider

1. Is emotional dysregulation primarily a limbic system or frontal lobe issue? What implications does your answer have for improving emotional management?

2. How do actors or dancers nonverbally convey emotions? Do we feel their emotion within our own bodies as we watch? How?

What's Your EQ, and How Can You Improve It?
Lecture 11

This lecture will introduce you to and deconstruct the idea of emotional intelligence. You will learn the behavioral strategies that people might use to regulate their emotions. You will learn about the science, as well as some of the pseudoscience, to determine if there are some important concepts that we can still use to address the biopsychosocial questions that we have about our health. If emotions play a role, can emotional intelligence deepen our understanding and even point to potential interventions?

What Is Emotional Intelligence?

- The four-branch model of emotional intelligence was originally developed by John Mayer and Peter Salovey in 1997 at Yale University. The four branches are as follows: Emotional intelligence is the ability to perceive emotion in the self and others; to use emotion, such as harnessing emotion, for a cognitive task; to understand and reason with emotion; and to regulate or manage emotion in the self and others.

- If we're using the four-branch model, we would use the Meyer-Salovey-Caruso Emotional Intelligence Test (MSCEIT) to measure emotional intelligence. This test is very similar to an IQ test. It is divided into many subscales because we have different emotional capacities—just as we have different intellectual capacities.

- An alternative is the BarOn Emotional Quotient Inventory (BarOn EQ-i®). This particular test probably taps a little bit more into dispositions, or personality.

- Furthermore, a much shorter, easier, and widely available self-report questionnaire was developed by Schutte. However, it is uncertain whether we have enough self-awareness to accurately assess and gauge our emotional intelligence.

- What does emotional intelligence predict? There's some science in this area, but there's also some pseudoscience. A lot of the research uses the MSCEIT, the test that tends to have better validity and reliability as a psychometric instrument.

- Low EQ, as measured by the MSCEIT, predicts more alcohol consumption and more drug use among college students. Low EQ also predicts less satisfying interpersonal relationships.

- Other studies have looked at emotional intelligence in the workplace. High emotional intelligence leads to better relationships with your peers as well as with your bosses. It means that you have a more positive mood while at work and better evaluations from your boss.

Changing Emotional Intelligence

- Can you change your emotional intelligence? It depends on how you define it. If you are of the persuasion that emotional intelligence is a personality trait, then personality, by definition, is not that changeable. You can learn some compensatory strategies, but you're probably stuck with what you were born with.

- If you see emotional intelligence as a collection of teachable skills and abilities, then you can absolutely increase your emotional intelligence. Think of it as a musical ability. Anyone can learn to play a musical instrument; some of us have more natural talent than others, but we can all practice and get better.

- James Gross at Stanford University wrote the textbook on emotion regulation. He has a few different research methodologies, but there is one that's most commonly used.

- Essentially, Gross hooks up a person to neurophysiologic equipment to measure muscle tension, heart rate, and blood pressure. Then, a mood is induced by showing a video, which is often grotesque. The subject has a physiologic response, and he's able to track that response.

- Gross may ask you to try to regulate your emotion in certain ways. He may put another person in the room or put your pet in the room to look at different ways that we can regulate the way we're feeling—so that we can turn that arousal back down.

- Emotion regulation can be extrinsic or intrinsic. Someone can change your emotional state, but it comes from an extrinsic place. Intrinsic emotional regulation is whatever strategies we're using inside of our heads or bodies to try to change our emotional state.

- Most of the adult research that James Gross and others have done focus on intrinsic emotion regulation. Even though we're not often aware of the emotion regulation that's going on, it happens all the time. Usually, the research looks at turning down negative emotional experiences—not turning them up.

- One strategy that people use to regulate their emotions is to change the situation, changing what they're exposed to. The second is distraction, or attentional deployment. (For example, when you're really angry, you count to 10.) The third category of strategies is about cognition, including rumination, savoring, and reappraisal. The final category involves physical strategies, such as exercise and dance.

- The consequences of regulation often depend on the social context. Sometimes it's appropriate to express emotions; sometimes it's not appropriate. For example, in certain contexts, it's completely appropriate to express your anger; in others, you probably don't want to express it because of the negative social consequences.

- Suppression, a common intrinsic emotion regulation strategy that's often used, comes at a cost. Suppression can be a form of avoidance. Suppression can also extend the effects of stress and intensify an emotion.

- We all use suppression, and sometimes suppression is appropriate. If you're not in the right setting to let it all come out, you want to suppress it, but eventually, you need to process and experience those feelings. However, expression doesn't necessarily equate with catharsis.

- There used to be literature about anger that talked about how important it is to express the anger. The literature in question would recommend interventions such as the following: When you're really, really angry, take a tennis racquet and beat your pillow with it to get all of that anger out of you.

- In fact, what that tends to do is amplify the physiologic arousal and make you more angry. There is a point at which physical exercise does cause you to be fatigued and anger might begin to diminish, but simple expression doesn't always work, and sometimes there are other regulation strategies that might help you get rid of that anger a little more effectively and quickly.

Generating Positive Emotions

- We probably don't need any help generating negative emotions, but what if we wanted to increase the percentage or proportion of positive emotions we have? Judith Moskowitz, at the University of California, San Francisco, has developed a robust research program. She has worked with very difficult, hard-to-reach populations that have many reasons to have negative emotions.

- For example, Moskowitz works with low-income women in Oakland who have recently been diagnosed with HIV. She brings those women into her lab and gives them a variety of interventions to see which of those can increase their level of positive emotions.

- The first intervention that she has found has worked is helping them to notice positive events that happen. This is an attention manipulation, probably because of survival. Maybe there's an evolutionary reason we're naturally drawn to notice negative things—we don't give the same attention to positive things.

- The second intervention has to do with savoring. When those positive things happen, she coaches them to ruminate about the positive.

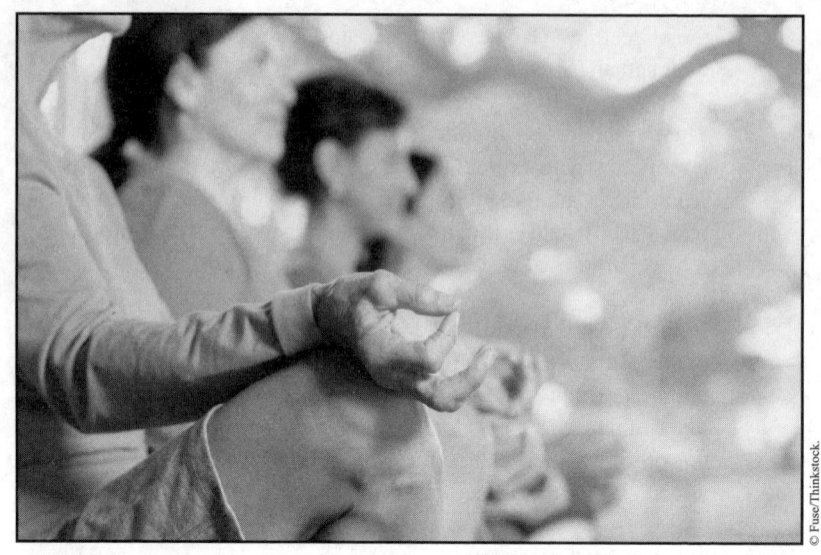

Mindfulness meditation has elements of somatic quieting, acceptance, and positive self-regard.

- The third intervention is gratitude. She has found that a very robust and effective way of ramping up positive affect is to have someone write a gratitude letter of what they're grateful for.

- The fourth intervention has to do with mindfulness and mindfulness meditation, which is a cognitive strategy that involves positive reappraisals focusing on personal strengths, and listing attainable goals—even if those are small steps so that you can have a "success" experience.

- The last intervention is acts of kindness. Sometimes you actually get more of a mood boost if you buy something for someone else instead of buying something for yourself.

- It can be argued that it is not really great to be so preoccupied with happiness, however. We need both positive and negative states; it's more about balance and how we can accurately respond to the world around us.

- However, in the realm of coping with chronic stressors, we usually don't need any help generating the negative. We might need some help generating the positive. Remember the cognitive behavioral therapy interventions and the types of cognitions (reappraisals and reframing).

- There's a new type of cognitive therapy called dialectic behavioral therapy. It's called "dialectic" because it's the balance between accepting versus wrestling with your thoughts.

- There are four modules of dialectic behavioral therapy. There is a mindfulness meditation component, which has its elements of somatic quieting, acceptance, and positive self-regard. There are also modules on interpersonal effectiveness, on emotion regulation, and on distress tolerance.

- There are actually a number of different acceptance-based behavioral therapies. Acceptance and commitment therapy, by Steve Hayes, is one of the most popular. In these therapies, it's not about wrestling with your thoughts; instead, it's about stepping back and realizing that a thought is just a thought. You don't need to do anything about it because you are not the problem.

Suggested Reading

Goleman, *Emotional Intelligence*.

Hayes, *Get Out of Your Mind and Into Your Life*.

Mayer, Salovey, and Caruso, "Models of Emotional Intelligence."

Pennebaker, *Opening Up*.

Remen, *Kitchen Table Wisdom*.

Seligman, *Authentic Happiness*.

———, *Flourish*.

———, *Learned Optimism*.

Questions to Consider

1. Does emotional intelligence always improve with age? What facilitates or impedes this learning process?

2. Should emotional intelligence be taught in schools? Should it be taught elsewhere? What teaching strategies would be most effective?

What's Your Type? Personality and Health
Lecture 12

In this lecture, you will learn about personality. You will learn about the aspects of personality that we believe are most closely related to health and disease. This lecture will also help you answer some fairly big questions: What is meant by personality? How do we measure it? How do we assess it? What kinds of personality types are there, and what do they mean? What is their utility? Are they evidence based? Then, the lecture will try to tie these typologies into health and discuss potential strategies to change or to compensate.

The History of Personality

- The earliest writings about personality were from Aristotle and his successor Theophrastus, who observed Greek citizens. From their observations, they were able to deduce a set of 30 different personality types, including things like the liar, the surly man, the tasteless man, and the flatter.

- Many centuries later, Galen proposed four temperament types based on the Hippocratic humors: Black bile was related to the melancholy personality; yellow bile was related to the choleric or angry person; phlegm was related to the phlegmatic person—or the calm, stolid person; and blood was related to the sanguine, warm-hearted, confident person.

- In the 18th century, we see the practice of phrenology, in which your personality and intelligence were assessed by people feeling the bumps on your head.

- Modern personality science tells us that there is some sort of hardwiring that gives us our initial interpersonal differences. However, those behaviors may change and adapt over time. There's a genetic, or "nature," component, but there also seems to be a developmental, or "nurture," component.

- World War I served as an impetus for the first scientifically developed personality test, but to develop a test, you have to have a concept of what it is you're trying to measure.

- Personality appears early in life, and it's resistant to change. It's a repetitive pattern, and it seems to be stable across situations. We weren't quite sure, though, what sorts of types we're supposed to be assessing.

- The first group personality test was the Army Alpha test, which was used in World War I as a way of filtering potential recruits. In the 1920s and 1930s, there was a lot of test development. This is when Meyers-Briggs was being developed and when Freud and Jung were developing their personality test.

- Later, behaviorism emerged and suppressed a lot of the personality science. Eventually, cognitive psychology emerged and reclaimed some of that personality science.

Personality Tests

- There are different scientific methods that have been used to derive some personality tests. One of the older ones is the 16 personality factors test (16PF), which was developed by Raymond Cattell in the 1940s and onward. Essentially, Cattell pulled out from the dictionary 4,500 adjectives that described interpersonal traits or possible personality traits. By looking at synonyms, he was able to reduce that list to 171.

- Then, he did a new procedure at the time called factor analysis on a brand new invention called the computer. He came up with a much-reduced list of 16—hence the 16 personality factors.

- In the late 1930s, the Minnesota Multiphasic Personality Inventory (MMPI) test was developed through a different methodology. The creators of this test were interested in clinical scales; they developed 10 different clinical scales. They have a total of 338 true/false items, and cleverly, they folded in a lie scale to see whether people are being truthful. Many people consider this a gold-standard personality test.

- There are other personality tests that are derived in other ways that aren't quite so scientific, although they may have a very long history behind them and a number of proponents. Examples of this type of test are Western astrology (Taurus or Gemini) and the Chinese zodiac (rat, dragon, or rabbit).

- Two newer, evidence-based typologies are the Five-Factor Model and personality types A, B, C, and D. The Five-Factor Model has come into its renaissance through the work of John Digman. The acronym for the five factors is OCEAN: openness, conscientiousness, extraversion, agreeableness, and neuroticism.

- In the 1980s, John Digman and colleagues developed a 240-item questionnaire called the NEO Five-Factor Personality Inventory, but more commonly, we use a much shorter inventory called the Big Five Inventory (BFI), which comes to us from Oliver John at the University of California, Berkeley.

- The BFI has 44 items. You either agree or you disagree with each statement, rating each on a scale of 1 to 5. Of course, they want to tap into all five of those factors across those 44 items, and eventually, you get a profile or score of where you stand on each of those.

Heritability of Personality
- From genetic studies, primarily from twin studies, we know that both heredity and environment are important in the expression of personality traits. If we look at the Big Five traits, openness to experience tends to be about 57 percent heritable, conscientiousness about 49 percent, extraversion about 54 percent, neuroticism about 48 percent, and agreeableness about 42 percent.

- The range is between 42 and 57 percent, so it looks to be about half nature and half nurture. This is important to because even though personality is resistant to change, half of it's not about genetics, so maybe there's hope.

- In terms of the Big Five personality traits, job performance is predicted by high conscientiousness and low neuroticism. Interpersonal conflicts are predicted by low openness to experience and high neuroticism. Low agreeableness and low conscientiousness are correlated with juvenile delinquency.

- Conscientiousness predicts better medical adherence, so it is related to improved health. Alternatively, neuroticism is linked with depression and other psychiatric disorders, which may in turn contribute to cardiovascular and other diseases. Furthermore, low agreeableness is related to anger and hostility, which are linked to cardiovascular disease.

Personality Styles
- The personality styles that we will discuss are simply called types A, B, C, and D, which actually have different scientists that have promoted them, have different tests that assess them, and are thought to be potentially related to different diseases.

- Type A is probably the most researched and the most familiar to the public. The type A person is someone who is very rushed, very impatient, and very competitive. The type A person is someone who wants to achieve more and more in less and less time. The type A person probably has a temper.

- The type B person is essentially the yin to the type A yang. The type B person is a laidback person who is not time pressured. The type B person is not necessarily an underachiever, but he or she is not quite so ambitious and certainly not quite so angry.

- Some people have made the claim that the "C" in type C stands for "cancer" and that maybe it's a personality type that predisposes us to cancer. Could that possibly be true?

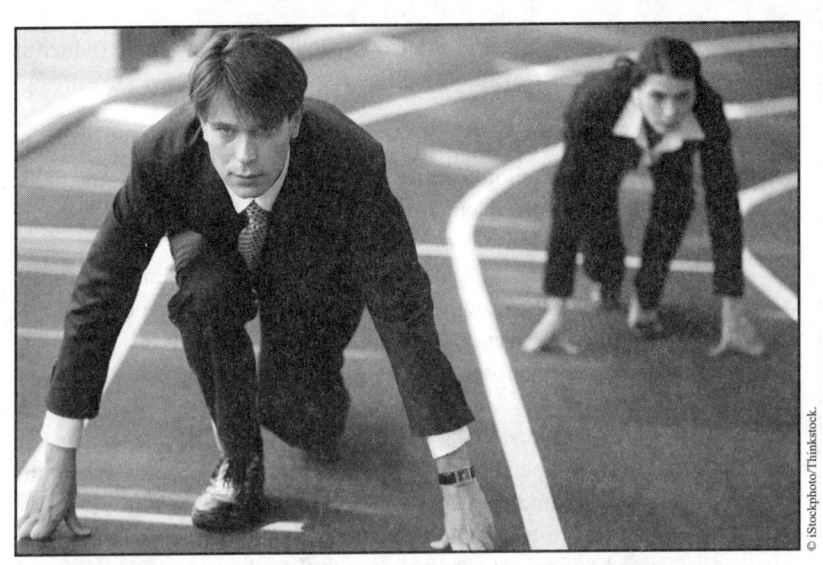

Competitiveness is one of the main personality traits of someone who is type A.

- The "D" in type D essentially stands for "distressed." The newest and most exciting area of research comes from researchers in the Netherlands and has been picked up by a number of cardiovascular researchers in the United States.

- The type A behavior pattern is described as a behavioral and emotional style marked by an aggressive, unceasing struggle to achieve more and more in less time, often in competition with others and other forces.

- The three key elements of type A behavior are as follows: easily aroused hostility, time urgency, and competitiveness. Of those three traits, it seems that hostility, especially easily aroused cynical hostility, is most closely associated with cardiovascular disease.

- Because hostility is the driving feature of linking the type A-B typology to health, it's unusual to see an assessment tool that measures this full personality type. Instead, we often see measures just of hostility, such as the Cook-Medley hostility scale (which is seen as a subset of the MMPI), or sometimes we see measures of cardiovascular reactivity.

- Type C is much more controversial than types A or B. Essentially, since the time of Galen, we've been trying to look at personality types that predispose people to cancer. A type C person suppresses their emotions and tends to deny strong emotional reactions. A type C person is more prone to developing hopelessness and helplessness. However, there's no proof that having a type C personality predisposes an individual to developing cancer.

- A type D person has a higher than average level of negative affectivity. A type D person is anxious and more prone to becoming depressed. In addition, a type D person doesn't turn to others for help. There are two components: negative affect, or emotions, plus social inhibition. The prevalence is thought to be as high as 20 percent to 35 percent of the population.

- If you're type A, B, C, or D or if you're high or low on the different dimensions of the Big Five, it is possible that you can change. By definition, personality traits are difficult to change. If we can't change the personality trait, however, maybe we can learn some compensatory strategies.

- Does a trait or tendency change, or is it just how we interpret or experience it internally? It might actually be a little bit of both. We know that we have neuroplasticity until death, so we can do all sorts of different rewiring. We don't know exactly where personality sits or if there's a critical window when we might be able to change it and if that window has passed or not.

Suggested Reading

Digman, "Personality Structure."

Larsen and Buss, *Personality Psychology*.

Valliant, *The Wisdom of the Ego*.

Questions to Consider

1. If personality is essentially fixed by late adolescence, can people really change? How can we know when to accept who we are versus struggle to be different?

2. Are there particular personality types that have good "chemistry" together? Do you find yourself surrounded by a particular kind of personality? Is this satisfying?

An Apple a Day—Behavior and Disease Prevention
Lecture 13

This lecture focuses on health-related behaviors. About 40 to 50 percent of premature morbidity and mortality are predicted by behavior. In this lecture, you will learn about some of the epidemiology around the leading causes of morbidity and mortality, specifically related to behaviors. This lecture will also address the question of why we do the things we do, and as a way to answer that question, you will learn about the neuroscience of behavior by looking at the neuroscience of addiction and habits.

Smoking

- Smoking is the top contributor to premature mortality. Recent surveys show that nearly 70 percent of current smokers would like to stop and 52.4 percent have tried to stop in the past year.

- Recent changes have been more about addressing the issue of secondhand smoking, or passive smoking. In fact, most states and counties now have laws that limit the places where smokers can smoke.

- When we talk about secondhand smoke, we're primarily worried about cardiovascular disease. There may be some increased risk of cancer, but most smokers die from heart attacks and not necessarily from cancer. We worry about the same for people who are passively inhaling secondhand smoke.

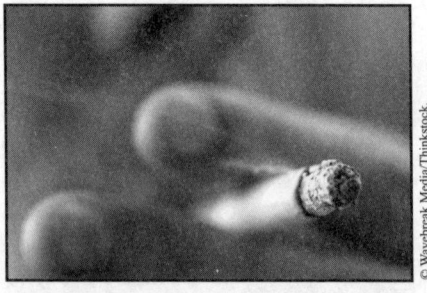

In the United States, about 20 percent of the population smoke cigarettes, causing about 450,000 deaths per year.

Nutrition and Exercise
- Most people are familiar with the food pyramid, which has been revised multiple times but was recently scrapped altogether. Today, we use MyPlate, which a simple graphic of a plate that is approximately divided into four different quadrants: a quarter for fruits, a quarter for vegetables, a quarter for protein, and a quarter for grains. Next to your plate sits a little cup, which is where the dairy goes.

- Unfortunately, people follow these recommendations only about two percent of the time. And in order to count as a person who followed the MyPlate recommendations, you only had to be 70 percent compliant.

- Nutrition is important in its own right, but we're also concerned about the number of calories that we're taking in. We're concerned about obesity and the health issues associated with it.

- The most commonly used measure of your weight is called the body mass index (BMI), which is calculated by taking your weight in kilograms divided by your height in meters squared.

- Some people have objected to the BMI, saying that it's not that precise of a measure. For example, if an individual has a lot of muscle mass—if they're an athlete or a weightlifter, for example—his or her BMI will actually place him or her in what's considered the overweight or even the obese category.

- An alternative is the waist-to-hip, which is measured by simply taking a measurement of those two parts of your body. The goal for men is that this ratio is less than 0.95, and the goal for women is less than 0.80.

- Using BMI, approximately 69 percent of men and women in the United States over the age of 20 are considered overweight. In order to be overweight, your BMI has to be over 25. In addition,

36 percent of Americans are considered obese, meaning that their BMIs are over 30.

- If we look at the rates of overweight and obese people over just the past two decades, they've been rising dramatically. And it's not just in adults; it's in children, too.

- How can we understand this interesting and worrying public health phenomenon? Is it about genetics? Probably not, but maybe we can make an epigenetic argument about it. Is it about lifestyle? Is it about our toxic food environment, where we have so much readily available fast food? It is probably all of the above or something else.

- It's not just about the calories that you take in; it's also about the calories that you burn off through physical activity and exercise. About 60 percent of U.S. adults don't exercise regularly, but 73 percent feel that they are in fair to excellent physical condition.

- Greater health benefits are associated with greater levels of activity, but it doesn't necessarily have to be intense or prolonged activity. Currently, the recommendation is to get approximately an hour of exercise per day nearly every day during the week. Most people find that unrealistic or a little bit daunting. However, any level of physical activity can potentially have health benefits.

Alcohol and Drug Use
- In the United States, 51 percent of adults are considered "regular drinkers," which is defined as having at least 12 drinks in the past year. In addition, approximately 8.7 percent use illicit drugs, 14 percent have used marijuana in the past year, and 3 percent have used prescription medications for nonmedical reasons.

- Rates of alcoholism for males run about 5 percent to 10 percent. For females, the rate is about 2 percent to 5 percent. About 25 to 40 percent of patients who occupy general hospital beds have alcohol problems. In addition, 70 percent of our prisoners have some form of a substance abuse problem.

- Substance and alcohol abuse are accountable for nearly one-third of all criminal justice costs. These types of abuse are related to 50 percent of all cases of child abuse and child neglect and to 80 percent of all fatal car crashes.

Biological Factors

- We hear a lot about genetics and obesity and about the genetics of alcoholism, for example. Many of these findings are taken from gene studies—studies of dizygotic or monozygotic twins who are either raised together or apart.

- For smoking, we heritability is approximately 44 percent. For obesity, heritability estimates range between 50 and 70 percent. For substance use disorders, the heritability rate is about 50 percent. This tells us that in terms of nature, it's about half, and in terms of nurture, it's about half.

- Evolutionarily, some would argue that we are wired to prefer salt and fat and, when we get what used to be those rare commodities, that we eat them as much as possible. Of course, we're in a different food environment today, and salts, fats, and sugars are readily available. Unfortunately, we still have those old impulses to overeat, and we end up eating much more than we actually need.

- As you get older, you get a little bit heavier. In fact, most people gain a few pounds per year, which can add up to a lot and have substantial effects on your health. The ratio of muscle mass to fat in your body affects your basal, or resting, metabolism rate.

- Some have estimated that 30 to 60 percent of exercise variance, meaning who exercises and who doesn't, is attributable to genetics. Think about the rewards and the punishment of exercise. One of the punishments of exercise is that you get very sore because you build up lactic acid in your muscles. The amount of lactic acid, or lactose, that a person generates is in part genetically determined.

- Another biological factor is low socioeconomic status and its relationship to chronic stress and fat. There is a link between hypercortisolemia and an individual putting on central obesity.

- People smoke to relieve stress. Eating stimulates dopamine, whose release helps us decrease our experience of stress. The same is true for alcohol and drugs, other ways to cope with stress. We have a lot of unhealthy habits as a way of trying to cope.

Psychological and Social Factors
- In addition to the biological reasons that we do the things we do, there are psychological and social factors. For example, we might look at education, income, and culture. We might look at societal pressures, marketing, advertising, and our "toxic food environment." We might also look at health policies and taxes and how those influence our behaviors.

- Lower education equals higher rates of smoking. Regardless of your level of education, everyone's rates of smoking have decreased since the 1970s. But the people who have benefited the most from antismoking campaigns are the people with the most education. The population we haven't really reached are those who are still smoking, which is often people with lower education.

- Does income predict substance use disorders—alcohol and drugs—beyond tobacco? That relationship is a little more complicated. In part, it depends on the drug, and in part, it depends on the route of administration.

- If you look at race and ethnicity, sticking with the example of smoking, we see by far the highest smoking rates in the American Indian and native Alaskan populations—rates of around 31 percent. The percentage for African Americans is about 21 percent while the percentage for Asians is only about 9 percent.

- Commercials, marketing, and advertisements are terrific at creating emotional ties to food. Just imagining foods like apple pie and lemonade probably stirs up some emotions for you. Supermarkets are masterful in how they manipulate our choices.

Suggested Reading

American Dietetic Association. *Complete Food and Nutrition Guide.*

Dunn, Andersen, and Jakicic, "Lifestyle Physical Activity Interventions."

Estabrook, Glasgow, and Dzewaltowski, "Physical Activity Promotion through Primary Care."

Fanning and O'Neill, *The Addiction Workbook.*

Kringelbach and Berridge, *Pleasures of the Brain.*

Questions to Consider

1. Can food really be an addiction similar to a drug? At what point does enjoyment of food become too much? How can you know?

2. Given that many people have multiple health behaviors they need to change, where should they start first? Should they try to fix them all at once?

Staying on the Wagon—Making Changes That Last
Lecture 14

In this lecture, you're going to explore the notion of long-term behavior changes—changes that stick. You will learn about some of the statistics on change rates. From the leading models of change, you will identify some core concepts—including self-control, self-discipline, motivation, and willpower—and look at what they really mean. The lecture will end by broadening the scope of interventions for behavior change to look at groups, communities, and even whole societies.

Realistic Expectations

- Many people have tried to lose weight, quit smoking, stop using substances, or stop drinking alcohol. There have been a number of different behavioral studies looking at each of these different behaviors independently, and a few recent studies have looked at multiple behavior changes at the same time.

- From these different behavioral studies, we're able to deduce four different key ingredients of successfully changing your behavior. The first is having realistic expectations and appropriate goals. The second is having an internal motivation, or a sense of will that you want to do it. The third is about core skills—knowing exactly what to do so that your new healthy behaviors become habits. Lastly, it's about having an achievable action plan.

- In addition to these four key ingredients, we know that support from your social circles—and even support from the environment—are critical ingredients.

- The first key ingredient is about realistic expectations or goals. If you set an unrealistic goal, you're simply setting yourself up for failure. It's okay to shoot high, but it's very unmotivating if month after month goes by and you haven't reached or achieved that goal.

- In general, goals should be SMART: specific, measurable, attainable, relevant, and timely.

Internal Motivation
- Motivation is sort of a tricky thing. It can be thought of in terms of stages of change, and there are particular interventions that might increase an individual's level of motivation. The term "motivation" can be defined as "the activation of goal-oriented behavior."

- Motivation can come from inside or from outside. In general, if you are intrinsically motivated, you're more likely to make behavioral changes that last.

- There are at least three things that determine motivation: having a sense of importance and value, having a sense of self-efficacy or self-confidence, and being in the appropriate social setting or context.

- We can make lists to help us see why it is important for us to change our behavior, but the problem is that we forget why things are so important. We become distracted and forget about our goal and values. We need to think of a way to keep these ideas fresh, to frequently revisit these values, and to remind ourselves of how important they might be.

- Self-efficacy is the belief that one is capable of performing in a certain manner to attain certain goals. Essentially, it's self-confidence. People with high self-efficacy are more likely to view difficult tasks as something to be mastered rather than something to be avoided. High self-efficacy predicts smoking cessation, physical exercise, dieting, condom use, dental hygiene, seat belt use, and even breast examinations.

- Our health-related behaviors are very much influenced by the people around us. We find our tribe, and the tribe has similar behaviors. Either you change your social circle, which is not so easy, or you give them clear instructions. They need to know about your goals and values and what they can do to help or support you.

- In terms of your social environment, it is important to remove temptations or triggers whenever possible. It's a process called stimulus control. If you're trying to limit the amount that you eat, either don't have those unhealthy, tempting foods in the house, or if you do eat those foods, make sure that you take out only the amount that you want to eat and put the rest of it away.

Core Skills
- Core skills can come from a number of different places. They can come from inside of you (motivation, or self-regulation). They can come from your inner circle of friends and family or perhaps even your medical providers. They might also come from your environment.

- In the 1960s and 1970s, Walter Mischel devised an experiment on self-regulation that has been called the marshmallow test. For this test, you sit a child down at a table and put a delicious marshmallow, maybe with a little bit of chocolate on top, on a plate in front of them.

- You tell the child, "If you want to eat that, you can eat it, or when I leave the room, if you can wait 5 or 10 minutes, I'll come back and you can have two marshmallows." There are many variants of this test, and the children use some hilarious strategies to resist temptation.

- From these experiments, Mischel found that the capacity for self-regulation starts to improve in four- and five-year-old children and that the capacity for self-regulation at that very young age can actually predict success in elementary school and high school and can even predict performance on the SATs.

- Self-regulation has a number of different elements. First, it's about self-observation. Before we can control or change something, we have to be able to gather data about ourselves. Then, there's self-evaluation. Once you have that data about yourself, what's the ruler that you're using? Are you above or below your goal? The third

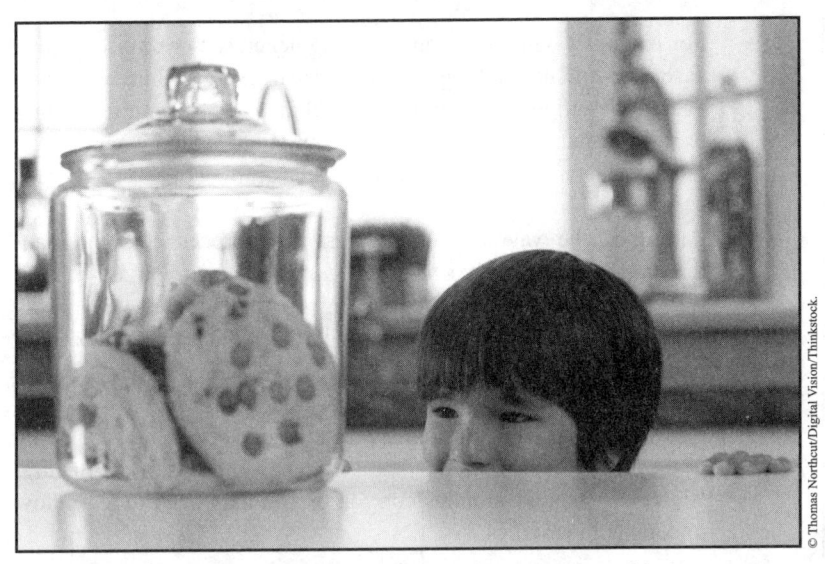

Our health-related behaviors, including being able to resist cookies, are very much influenced by the people around us.

part is self-reaction. Based on how you're doing, do you reward or punish yourself?

- Willpower is a very slippery construct. We'd like to think that we're completely in control of our behavior, but we know that there are all sorts of different influences.

- There are a number of recent and very interesting books on willpower. For example, in Roy Baumeister's book, he talks about self-control as a limited resource that can be drained through exertion, almost like a muscle. If you're repeatedly using that muscle, the muscle becomes fatigued and you can't use it as much.

- Stress—the fight-or-flight response—drains our willpower. When we get less sleep, we have less willpower. Hopefully, there are things that we can do behaviorally to increase our willpower.

- For example, willpower can be strengthened with exercise. In this case, we are not talking about physical exercise but willpower exercise: setting realistic goals, realizing when you're getting exhausted, and then removing temptation—waiting until you recover. The next time, you go a few steps further.

- Falling off the wagon is actually part of the process. It's important that you not be harshly self-critical. In fact, when you are harshly self-critical of yourself for messing up, it increases your stress response, which decreases your willpower. Instead, you need to have some flexibility.

- You should also include reflection and adaptations of your goals if they should prove unrealistic. You may need some structural strategies, such as stimulus control, or you may need to learn how to cope with cravings.

- In terms of strategies from the environment, fear-based appeals have some limited support. Positive role models and positive examples can be helpful. From the new field of behavioral economics, there are a number of different strategies that may help us gain the system just a little bit. The effectiveness of things like cigarette taxes is an example.

Action Plans

- The last of the key ingredients is about achievable action plans. We want our goals to be realistic, and we want our action plan to involve having our resources in place. We want a start date. We want to share plans with our social circle. We need regular assessments. We need to anticipate obstacles. Expect setbacks and lapses.

- We may need regular consultations with a health-care provider or a health coach. Paradoxically, being structured may actually free us from our impulses.

- Recall that 40 percent of premature mortality is attributable to behavior. Change can be very difficult, but it's not impossible.

Habits can be useful, but they can also be very difficult to change and sometimes unhealthy. We should turn them to our advantage.

- Remember that the four pathways—the autonomic nervous system, the HPA axis, immunology, and epigenetics—are all at play even though we're talking about behavior.

Suggested Reading

Baumeister and Tierney, *Willpower*.

Duhigg, *The Power of Habit*.

Dunn, Andersen, and Jakicic, "Lifestyle Physical Activity Interventions."

Estabrook, Glasgow, and Dzewaltowski, "Physical Activity Promotion through Primary Care."

Fanning and O'Neill, *The Addiction Workbook*.

McGonigal, *The Willpower Instinct*.

Miller and Rollnick, *Motivational Interviewing*.

Prochaska, Norcross, and DiClemente, *Changing for Good*.

Rollnick, Mason, and Butler, *Health Behavior Change*.

Questions to Consider

1. If the capacity for self-regulation is measurable as early as elementary school and predicts success decades later, what can parents do to improve their impulsive child's abilities?

2. Have you ever permanently changed an important health behavior? What strategies did you use that worked (or didn't work)?

Ease the Burn—Modern-Day Stress and Coping
Lecture 15

Stress is often the most common element that helps us understand how the outside gets inside. This lecture offers a closer look at how stress affects our bodies, and it explores what we can do about it. In this lecture, you will learn about stress as the integration of biology, cognition, behavior, social factors, and emotional factors. You will also learn about particular terms that help us define stress and coping and how we might measure them. Finally, you will be exposed to a menu of different stress-management options.

Stress

- An important assumption is that just because you're stressed, it doesn't mean that you're not coping well. In fact, some stress may actually be good. A little bit of stress—just the right amount—can actually help improve our performance.

- Another assumption is that coping is a developmental phenomenon. Recall some of the biggest stressors earlier in your life, such as the very first loss of a love or the first death that you experienced. Think about how much you've grown and how your coping strategies and mechanisms have changed.

- Stress is the biological, psychological, emotional, behavioral, and social responses to a stressor, which is the real or imagined event that sets things off. Coping is the set of adaptive or maladaptive responses meant to help us deal with the stress response.

- It's true that two people can have the exact same stressor but very different stress responses. One stress response may be very strong and intense while the other may not be present at all. The difference is not just about biology; it's also about cognition.

- With stress and coping, it's about appraisals. There are two kinds of appraisals: primary appraisals and secondary appraisals. Primary appraisal is about the stressor itself: Does it matter? Is it big? What are the outcomes? Should I care? The second kind of appraisal is about coping and about the amount of resources that you have.

- If a stressor occurs, you believe it's a really big deal (primary appraisal), and you don't have any resources to cope (secondary appraisal), then you're going to have a fairly robust stress response.

- All stressors are not created equal. Stressors can be classified as either challenges or threats. Both are arousing, but it's only the threats that we worry about in terms of our health. Stressors can also be acute or chronic. In terms of our health, we're much more worried about chronic stressors.

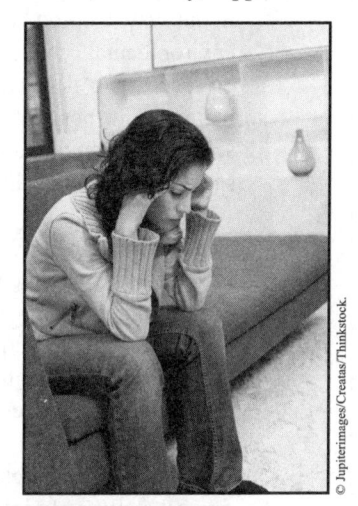

Stress is the integration of biology, cognition, behavior, social factors, and emotional factors.

- Events that are negative, that are uncontrollable, that have more ambiguity, or that are novel are most likely going to increase the level of your stress response—especially if you are already overloaded. It's important to remember that good events, such as moving to a new city, can also be stressful.

- Self-report, or a questionnaire, is probably the most common method of measuring stress. There are also performance tasks, such as the Trier Social Stress Test, or different physiologic measures, such as cardiovascular reactivity

Coping

- Hopefully, coping is our response to whatever stressors might be in our way. Coping has five primary goals: to decrease the harmful environmental conditions and increase prospects for recovery or success; to help us tolerate adjustments to negative events; to maintain our positive self-image, self-confidence, self-esteem, and self-regard; to maintain emotional equilibrium; and to continue our satisfactory relationships with others.

- The early coping models didn't call it "coping"; instead, they called it "psychological defenses." The father of psychoanalysis, Sigmund Freud, talked about defense mechanisms, which were all about the overtaxed ego and about repressing internal desires from your id—the strategies that were used by the unconscious mind to make unacceptable impulses acceptable.

- The period of time between the 1940s and 1960s was the heyday of ego psychology. Individuals such as Anna Freud, Sigmund Freud's daughter, and Alfred Adler, one of Freud's students believed that it's not just about the internal world—it's also about the external world. The goal was to strengthen the ego.

- The id is our primal impulses; the ego is our conscious mind; and the superego is our internalized parent, or our conscience. The central functions of the ego were typically seen as things like reality testing, impulse control, and judgment—what we would probably now call system-two thinking.

- In the 1960s, during the so-called cognitive revolution, Aaron Beck was developing cognitive behavioral therapy, but a number of psychologists were also beginning to look inside at cognition and to look at the brain.

- Richard Lazarus was one such psychologist. Along with a graduate student, Susan Folkman, he developed what was called the cognitive-transactional model of coping. This is where the primary and secondary appraisals come from.

- Coping can be divided into two categories: problem-focused coping and emotion-focused coping. Problem-focused coping is essentially a set of strategies that directly impacts the stressor. Fro example, studying for a test is a problem-focused coping strategy.

- Emotion-focused coping doesn't do much about the stressor, but it improves our emotional state so that maybe we're more able to cope at some point in the future. Calling a friend, reading a novel, or going to a movie doesn't change the stressor, but it probably changes your emotional state.

- The most successful people at coping are those who are able to find just the right balance between problem-focused coping and emotion-focused coping. The balance depends on the stressor. If the stressor is something that is controllable and changeable, you probably want to do a little more problem-focused coping. If the stressor is something that you absolutely cannot change or that changes only with great difficulty, you probably need a fair dose of emotion-focused coping. Of course, it's also about being flexible. If one strategy doesn't work, then change.

- One way to measure coping is to use the Ways of Coping Questionnaire, which was developed by Folkman and Lazarus. This is a 66-item questionnaire that divides coping into eight different categories. It is very much rooted in their cognitive-transactional model of coping.

- The eight categories of coping are as follows: confrontive coping, distancing, self-controlling, seeking social support, accepting responsibility, escape-avoidance, planful problem solving, and positive reappraisal.

- In general, it looks like escape-avoidance coping tends to be the least successful form of coping, followed by distancing. The most successful, depending on the stressor, are planful problem solving and seeking social support.

Stress Management

- While the meaning of the term "stress management" is obvious, the most effective strategies might not be so obvious.

- Stress management entails the need to develop the skills of acute appraisals—an optimal selection of coping strategies based on controllability, resources, and importance.

- Essentially, we first need to be aware that we're stressed and that we need to do something, and then we will select both cognitive and behavioral strategies from a long menu of possibilities, keeping in mind what Folkman tells us about the healthiest ways of coping and remembering that what we'll choose depends on our own capacities, interest, time, and skill.

- The items on this menu can be divided into two categories: cognitive strategies and behavioral strategies. Most simply, on the cognitive side is distraction. Behavioral interventions include seeking social supports, which may be a dispositional factor, and balancing the activities—what you have to do and what you want to do—in your life.

- Emotion-focused coping is another way to alleviate stress and put you in a good mood. This might include things like physical activity or exercise.

- Mindfulness meditation typically focuses on paying attention to your breath, for example. As you pay attention, you get some somatic quieting. Some of the common elements across all of the different kinds of meditation are relaxation, acceptance, and concentration.

- Research shows that meditation can reduce stress, the experience of pain, depression, and anxiety and can result in improvements in quality of life.

Resilience
- Resilience, which is part of stress and coping, is defined as when a powerful biological and/or environmental risk factor does not produce the expected negative outcome. Somehow the individual, despite all odds, has a high subjective well-being even in the presence of adversity.

- There has been a lot of research looking at the predictors or features of resilience. There need to be environmental buffers, such as an enriched environment or the support of adults or adult surrogates. There needs to be a place of refuge.

- There may also be cognitive or personality factors that can be helpful. In terms of learned helplessness and attributional style, a child who is able to realize that whatever happened is not his or her fault, that the situation is going to change, and that it has to be different somewhere else is better able to be resilient.

- It might also be about temperament. For example, children who are more extroverted, affectionate, and outgoing tend to elicit more social support.

Suggested Reading

Davis, Eshelman, and McKay, *The Relaxation and Stress Reduction Wookbook*.

Folkman and Moskowitz, "Coping."

Kabat-Zinn, *Full Catastrophe Living*.

Lazarus and Folkman, *Stress, Appraisal, and Coping*.

Lehrer, Woolfolk, and Sime, *Principles and Practice of Stress Management*.

Martz and Livneh, *Coping with Chronic Illness and Disability*.

McEwen, "Stress, Adaptation, and Disease."

Reivich and Shatte, *The Resilience Factor*.

Remen, *Kitchen Table Wisdom*.

Salzberg, *Loving-Kindness*.

Satterfield, *A Cognitive-Behavioral Approach to the Beginning of the End of Life*.

———, *Minding the Body*.

Snyder, *Coping*.

Questions to Consider

1. Given the dramatically different outcomes for the men in the longitudinal Grant Study of Harvard students (1937), what could the university have done to better equalize the students' abilities to cope and succeed?

2. Is the Eastern spirituality often attached to meditation necessary to enjoy its beneficial health effects? What might you lose or gain by carving it out?

The Iceberg—Visible and Hidden Identity
Lecture 16

The focus of this lecture is identity, which is defined as the characteristic determining who or what a person or thing is. Elements or characteristics of identity include race, ethnicity, gender, age, sexual orientation, physical attributes, personality, political affiliations, religious beliefs, professional identities, and so on. This lecture will address the following questions: What are the elements of identity? How do we perceive, change, and build identity? How does identity affect our health?

Individual Identity

- We belong to multiple groups at the same time. We may hold some traits more central to our identity than others, but not everyone holds that same value system. In fact, what we value the most might change as we grow older. This overlapping, interconnected aspect of identity is called intersectionality—the intersection of those different elements of our identity.

- Our identities are somewhat fluid. Although some characteristics are stable—including height, skin color, and maybe even some personality traits—our identity develops over time.

- There are a number of different stage theories of identity development, mostly concerned with race, that range from starting with denial to immersion to autonomy and eventually to integration. In short, we try to find our tribe while being able to connect with and to understand others. Our tribe shares the same culture.

- A culture is the collage of language, beliefs, traditions, codes of conduct, rules, memberships, and health beliefs that guide our daily lives. Our culture influences our tastes, food choices, sensations of pain and pleasure, and even how we love.

- Like identity, we can belong to many cultures at the same time; however, we can't necessarily be competent in all of them. In fact, belonging to a culture doesn't mean you're competent or fully understand that particular culture.

Identity Development

- In order for identity to develop, we need three things to happen: categorization, identification, and comparison.

- Sue Estroff and her social medicine colleagues at the University of North Carolina at Chapel Hill have done a lot of research on categorization. They tell us that it's a natural human inclination to make sense of things, to draw connections, and to look for relationships. That's just how we think.

- Part of the process is essentially sorting people and places into categories that either we or our cultures have created. Categories are complex, and some of the most complex categories are often central to our identity.

- Race is defined as a classification system used to categorize humans into large and distinct populations or groups by anatomical, cultural, ethnic, genetic, geographical, historical, linguistic, religious, or social affiliation. Essentially, race is our attempt to categorize, or sort people into categories, based on their skin color and a very small set of physical characteristics.

- There is a raging debate between geneticists and anthropologists about whether race is a biological construct. Could you look at someone's genome, for example, and determine what their race is without looking at where they are from or at their ancestors? Anthropologists correctly point out that there's often more genetic variation within one particular race than between the races.

- In addition to categorization, identification and comparison are the other two aspects of identity development.

- When we make categories, we open the door to making judgments. How we judge depends on how we self-identify: We tend to positively reappraise people who are in our in-group and tend to devalue people in another category—people in the out-group.

- How do we identify or join a group? There's a similar model to the biopsychosocial model called the social-ecological model that talks about social spheres of influence. Think about concentric circles, with individuals in the center, then their significant other and maybe their family is in the next circle, and then their neighbors, communities, countries, and the globe. All of these influences may be present at any particular time.

- In the process of identity formation, people look for similarities and differences between themselves and others, maybe with profound psychological consequences.

- Our identity changes over time. Part of young adulthood is deciding who your tribe is. As we start connecting with a particular group of people, we start to minimize our differences and maximize our

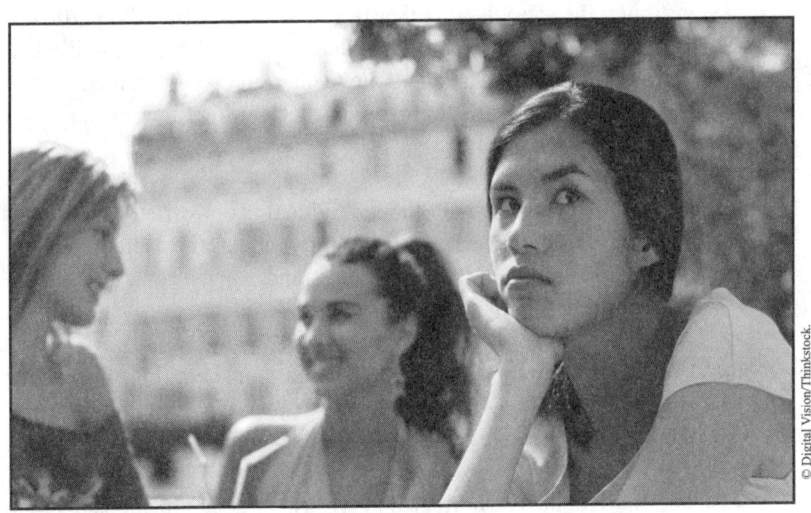

Many teenagers struggle with defining their identity.

similarities. Cognitive distortions—specifically, generalizations about the in-group being terrific and out-group being not so great—start to kick in.

- Your identity affects your self-concept, sense of value, and sense of self-esteem. It also affects your sense of perceived control. There is a hierarchy, or ladder of power, in society. Sometimes you can choose and sometimes others choose for you where are you on that ladder based on what your identity is.

- Being the recipient of stereotypes, bias, discrimination, or prejudice may be due to either hidden or visible identity. Visible identity is, for example, an individual who is stereotypically African American, including skin color and hair. Hidden identity is, for example, someone who is Jewish. There may be a cost of hiding if we don't make our hidden identity visible.

Cognitive Biases

- Stereotype threat refers to being at risk of confirming a self-characteristic, a negative stereotype about one's group. For example, the stereotype is that if you are a member of a particular race, then you're not going to do very well in school. An individual of this race does not have to believe the stereotype, but the fact that he or she knows that stereotype exists can affect him or her when taking an exam.

- Regardless of whether the individual is worried about not doing well on the exam or is angry about the stereotype, it's taking up some cognitive resources, and it may actually create a self-fulfilling prophesy.

- Cognitive shortcuts are neither good nor bad, but they have consequences. They're there for a reason, and sometimes we use them too much while other times we use them too little.

- The first cognitive shortcut that we use is generalizations—which aren't necessarily bad. We make generalizations all the time.

We look for patterns, trying to save mental processing energy. This is all about system-one thinking. It's efficient and helps us see connections.

- The second cognitive shortcut is about positive, or optimistic, bias. Most of us have a self-serving bias in which we pretty much see ourselves as above average in all sorts of different things. This is probably our psychological defense mechanisms.

- Of course, if self-serving bias is used too much, then we have an unrealistic sense of who we are and what we're able to accomplish, and maybe we don't see our weaknesses or work to improve ourselves. It does build pride. It gives us a sense of belonging and self-esteem, but it may come at a cost if used too much.

- Another common cognitive bias is the devaluation of the out-group. This happens all the time. We increase our opinions of our in-group and decrease our opinions of and maybe even dehumanize individuals in an out-group. This probably eases guilt from competition between those two groups.

- The labels and frames we use may subtly or not so subtly affect our opinions, judgments, and generalizations about others.

- We can't get away from cognitive biases and system-one thinking, but we can be explicit and open in reflecting about our identities and the groups that we belong to. We can be careful when we're evaluating ourselves—and particularly careful when we're evaluating our out-group.

- It's critical that we leave our comfort zones and interact with people that maybe we're not especially drawn to so that we get to know them as individuals and not as a generalization or stereotype.

- Diversity in all of its many different forms can be vexing, but it can also be quite valuable. When combined together, the different perspectives, different ways of thinking, and different life histories may cause us to see things that we wouldn't have seen if we only hang around people that are similar to us.

Identity and Health

- The 2002 Institute of Medicine report called *Unequal Treatment* distinguishes between health disparities, which are differences in the prevalence or outcomes of disease, and health-care disparities, which is when care is unequally provided to two people even though they have the same disease.

- For example, the life expectancy for a black man in the United States is about the same as a poor farmer in Bangladesh. What's going on? We should think about chronic stress, cardiovascular reactivity, and allostatic load. We also need to think about social factors.

- Most people that go into medicine or health care want to help other people—they don't want to provide unequal care. Health-care disparities are about implicit biases and how implicit biases can sometimes be made manifest, particularly if you're tired, rushed, or multitasking.

- When we try to measure implicit bias, we find that we all have biases, regardless of our background, race, or gender. Our task is to be aware of them and do what we can to change them.

Suggested Reading

Geronimus, Hicken, Keene, and Bound, "'Weathering' and Age Patterns of Allostatic Load Scores among Blacks and Whites in the United States."

Helms, "Black and White Racial Identity."

Institute of Medicine, *Unequal Treatment*.

King and Straus, et al, *The Social Medicine Reader*.

Marx, Ko, and Friedman, "The 'Obama Effect.'"

Steele and Aronson, "Stereotype Threat and the Intellectual Test Performance of African-Americans."

Stone, Lynch, Sjomeling, and Darley, "Stereotype Threat Effects on Black and White Athletic Performance."

Questions to Consider

1. Why is it that explicit ideologies and actual behavior often differ? How can we more closely align our behavior and our explicit beliefs?

2. Under what circumstances are implicit biases most likely to emerge? What can we realistically do to diminish bias in those situations?

Ties That Bind—Relationships and Health
Lecture 17

This lecture focuses on social support. In this lecture, you will take an in-depth look at relationships and, specifically, the support that your social connections can provide—support both given and received. You will learn about the key characteristics of social support, and you will review the research linking social support to health. In addition, you will be exposed to some of the questions that research on social support has yet to provide answers to.

Sociobiology and Social Support

- Sociobiology is a field of scientific study that is based on the assumption that social behavior has resulted from evolution, and it attempts to explain and examine social behaviors, such as relationships, mating, competing for resources, and fighting to survive. It's all about wanting to pass on your genes to procreate.

- Social support has been conceptualized in a number of different ways. In fact, it's a notoriously slippery concept to define and even harder to measure.

- The most commonly used definition of social support is that it is the perception and actuality that one is cared for, has assistance available from other people, and is part of a supportive social network. These supportive resources can be emotional, such as nurturance; tangible, such as financial assistance; informational, such as someone giving you advice; or companionship, such as having a sense of belonging.

- Research studies use the term "social support," but they also talk about social integration, social connectedness, and social support networks—each of which is a slightly different way of looking at the same complex, multifaceted concept.

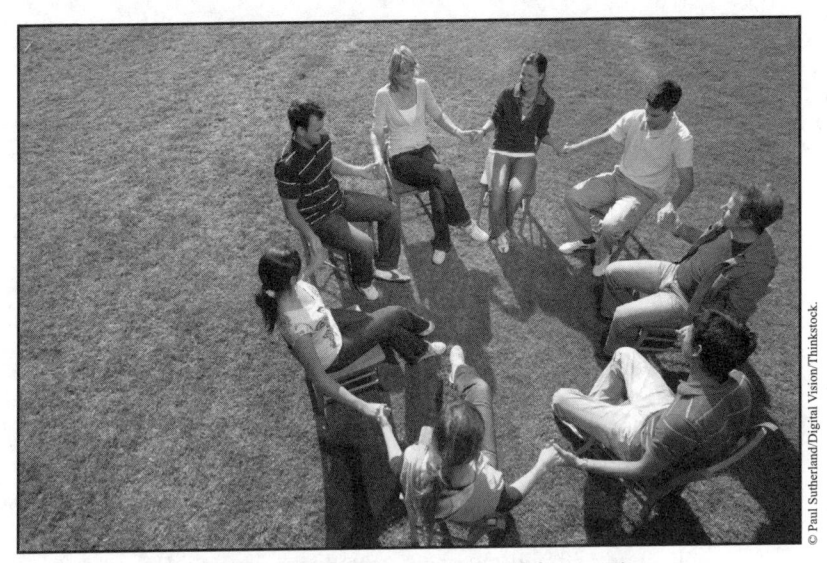

People in support groups both give and receive social support.

- If you wanted to measure or characterize your social support system, you would first look at the size, which is simply the number of individuals that you could turn to for help—any sort of help.

- Next, you might want to look at the density, which is essentially distance. Of those people that you can turn to for social support, how many are just a few miles away versus on the other side of the country? Just because of that distance, it makes the social support a little more difficult to access, and it may even limit the kinds of support that they're able to provide.

- The next thing you might look at is the diversity of your social supports. Are all of them approximately just like you—men or women of the same age and in the same profession? What's the diversity of your social support network?

- Next, we would look at reciprocity. Is there a two-way street between you and your social supports? Do you give as much support as you receive?

- Of course, this goes beyond the familial. Sometimes our families are supportive, and sometimes we need to strike out on our own and find a proxy family, a nonbiological family composed of friends and neighbors.

- There are four different kinds of support, and each of these is important. As you're thinking about the health of your social support network, you want to think about the structure, but you also need to determine whether or not you have all four kinds of these supports readily available.

- The first kind of support is emotional support. This is someone who will listen and will give you a shoulder to cry on. We need those emotional support providers.

- The second functional characteristic is informational support. Sometimes we need people to bounce ideas off of; we need people to provide advice.

- The third functional characteristic is tangible, or practical, support. This is someone who might not be great at emotional support or who might not be a good problem solver or advice giver, but he or she can at least help you cook dinner or clean up your house.

- The fourth characteristic has to do with companionship or belonging. It's difficult to feel isolated. This isn't the individual that you necessarily tell all of your problems to. This is someone who is willing and able to spend time with you. This is that person who calls for no reason, and you feel connected.

- Social support is about both perceived and actual support. Often, those two aren't quite the same. Perceived social support has a much stronger relationship to our health than any actual objective measures of social support.

- Is it about giving support or receiving support? Hopefully, there is some degree of reciprocity between you and your social supports. Most research is on receiving social supports. Sometimes too much caregiving and having to provide too much support can be difficult on the support giver.

- Sources of social support include significant others, family, and friends. Although you may see greater levels of intimacy in a romantic relationship, that doesn't have to be the case. Emotional closeness is often more about shared life experiences. It's just about support.

- In terms of the four functions of support, a pet or an animal might be able to provide emotional support—probably not so much in the way of advice, problem solving, or tangible support (although guide dogs and therapy dogs can certainly be helpful in a very practical and tangible way). They certainly could provide companionship, a feeling of belonging or being connected to another living thing. In fact, pets might even outperform humans in some contexts.

Social Support and Health
- What's the evidence that links social support to health? Behavior is responsible for approximately 40 percent of premature mortality. Smoking, diet, exercise, and obesity are at the top of that list.

- Our social networks—our tribe, culture, and family and friends—very much influence our health-related behaviors. Your social support networks are going to influence both your unhealthy and healthy behaviors.

- Lower social support is related to greater cognitive impairment and disability in adults. We're not quite sure of the mechanisms, but we think that it might be through health-related behaviors or medication adherence.

- In the Whitehall II study, a longitudinal study of British civil servants, marital status and social network scores predicted all-cause mortality for men. However, didn't hold true for women.

- Particularly impressive results have been found in the domain of cardiovascular disease. Specifically, research has found that social support equals a better chance at survival after a heart attack.

- In the Mended Hearts study, researchers used peer counseling and social support before patients went in to have cardiac bypass grafts. They found that people who had peer counseling and social supports actually had a better outcome after surgery—both psychiatrically and in terms of the medical outcome.

- Greater perceived support, especially perceived availability of emotional support, has been found to predict lower mortality risk among women with breast cancer. In addition, during pregnancy, greater perceived and received social support are linked to fewer labor complications and better birth outcomes.

- L. F. Griffith shows us that hemoglobin A1C, or a long-term measure of how well your blood sugar is controlled, was predicted by social support, but only during times of high stress. Social support wasn't related when stress was low, which makes sense.

- In a similar study by B. F. Erickson that looked at newly diagnosed type 2 diabetics, fasting blood glucose was lower in men with high perceived social support. However, this didn't seem to work in women.

Unanswered Questions
- The question of gender is vexing. It's easy to assume that women are just better at giving social support than men, but is that fair?

- An alternate hypothesis might be that men are just sicker and die earlier, so they have more room to improve. Another hypothesis might be that women have more relationships in general than men, so what they get from their husband is less unique and less valuable.

- In addition, there might be some sort of unique biologic effect. The interplay between estrogen and oxytocin could provide an answer, but this is still unknown.

- What are the health benefits of providing support? Some suggest that there are benefits of altruism, of helping another person, but other studies tell us that caregiving can be very stressful and actually damaging to your health.

- What about the effects of a negative relationship, a relationship that's full of conflict, compared to being socially isolated? We don't really know which is worse for your health.

- What about the importance of social support at different stages in your life? Does it matter more as a young adult, middle aged, or as an older adult? Again, we're not quite sure.

- There are a few different models that might help us understand how social support is related to health, but we're not quite sure what's right.

Suggested Reading

Brooks, *The Social Animal*.

King and Straus, et al, *The Social Medicine Reader*.

Nuon, "Phaly's Story."

Remen, *Kitchen Table Wisdom*.

Uchino, *Social Support and Physical Health*.

Questions to Consider

1. Are introverts more likely to have social support deficits? Why, or why not? How might social support development strategies differ for an extrovert versus an introvert?

2. Are individualistic societies, such as American society, trading social support for greater individuality? Is there a way we can have both?

Building Bridges—Intimacy and Relationships
Lecture 18

In this lecture, you will learn about intimacy, conflict, and strengthening social support networks. You will learn about the importance—the quantity and the quality—of relationships. You will also learn about the challenges of building intimacy. In addition, you will learn strategies for communication and for conflict resolution. At the end of the lecture, you will learn about ways to identify and manage anger and ways to cultivate empathy.

Building Relationships

- In modern times, families are more dispersed than ever before. We're electronically connected, but we're geographically distant. Our education, jobs, and responsibilities just push us further away from our families of origin.

- We may need to think about relationship building. This could be about quantity (just the body count) or quality (how many people are in your inner versus outer circle). It might be about the types of support, reciprocity, relationship maintenance, communication, conflict resolution, or deepening intimacy.

- When thinking about relationship building, consider whether you need to add new people (quantity). What's the right number? We really don't know. From most of the research, it looks like you need at least one confidant, or close friend who will be there for you anytime you pick up the phone. In other research, it looks like having two or maybe three social supports is even better. From a practical standpoint, it makes sense not to put all of your eggs in one basket.

- What about quality? What about the types of support that we have available? You need to ensure that you have adequate amounts of each type of support: informational, practical, emotional, and companionate. When you need support, it makes sense to identify in your mind whether you need emotional, informational, practical, or companionate support and then reach out to the right person.

- Of course, quality is also about intimacy and closeness. It's not that you need to have lots of people within your inner circle, because what might feel like intimacy to one person might feel completely smothering to another person. There's no right number of people to be in an inner circle.

- Intimacy is about your prior life events—your family and relationship history. Of course, it's also about communication and emotional skills. Each of us needs to look at our own personal inventory and make an assessment: Do we have sufficient intimacy? It's really about your perception.

- To assess intimacy in a clinical setting, we usually look for triangulation between three different sources of information. First, we'll give individuals self-report questionnaires, for example, to a husband and a wife. These often include perceptions about their life, finances, sex lives, children, and all sorts of other things. It's their perceptions of how things are now versus ideally how they would like them to be.

- Second, we interview each member of that couple separately, because sometimes they will tell us things individually that they might not if the other person is in the room.

- Third, we interview and observe them together. We get a sense of their communication style with one another and of their dynamics as a couple. From this, we can develop a working formulation of how best to help the couple.

- There are a number of different inventories that are available to measure intimacy. The most commonly used are the relationship closeness inventory, which can be about friendships or romantic relationships; and the PREPARE/ENRICH assessment tool, which is often used for premarital counseling.

- In terms of developing intimacy, time is our greatest gift. It's about shared activities and life events. It's about the diversity of those life events, in terms of having a mixed number of events. It's about shared struggles and challenges. Often, successfully working through conflicts brings people closer to one another.

- Intimacy is also about allowing yourself to take risks, to be vulnerable, and to create trust—even if it means that sometimes you might be let down. It means that you're good at communicating and understanding the needs of another person, but it also means that you are aware of your own needs and are able to ask that those needs are met.

- Intimacy means that we need to develop what's called interdependence, relying on one another and knowing that the sum total makes you each a better person.

Conflict and Conflict Management
- Conflict is probably one of the key ingredients to building intimacy. The most common sources of couples' conflict tend to fall into four categories: money, sex, children, and religion.

- We all have conflicts. Some of us express them while others suppress them. If they're suppressed, they sometimes come out in all sorts of interesting and unhelpful ways.

- When we think about conflict, there are emotional responses—biologic and physiologic arousal—especially anger and resentment. There are, of course, cognitive elements as well, including appraisal and how much importance we assign to it. There is also a behavioral component, which might include withdrawal, yelling, or quietly stewing.

- Relationships are potent triggers for automatic thoughts and emotions. Just as we have habits of mind, we have habits of the heart, including withdrawing or becoming competitive. Know what your habits of mind are and know how they get expressed within your relationship.

- What are some steps of conflict management? We need to gather data about ourselves, including self-reflection as well as external circumstances. We need to do some reality testing. As our emotional arousal goes up, our accuracy actually goes down, so it might be a good idea to get feedback from another person or cool off before we make decisions.

- We also need to make a diagnosis of the situation. What sorts of dynamics are going on? We need to develop an action plan and communicate that action plan. Then, review and reflect after the conflict to see if things have indeed been solved.

- There are many different methods to manage conflict, and there are all sorts of models of couples' therapy that can be helpful. The DESC method—describe, emote, specify, and consequences—essentially gives you a structured formula for communicating about conflict.

- *Getting to Yes*, a book from Harvard Business School, was first published in 1981 by Roger Fisher and William Ury. They focused on principled negotiation, or finding acceptable solutions by determining which needs are fixed and which are flexible. They also suggest having ready a BATNA (best alternative to negotiated agreement), which is essentially a backup plan.

Communication Skills
- Of course, miscommunication happens a lot. In fact, there are dramatic differences in the way that men and women communicate. In qualitative studies that have watched men and women in conversations, it seems that men spend about two-thirds of social conversations talking about themselves.

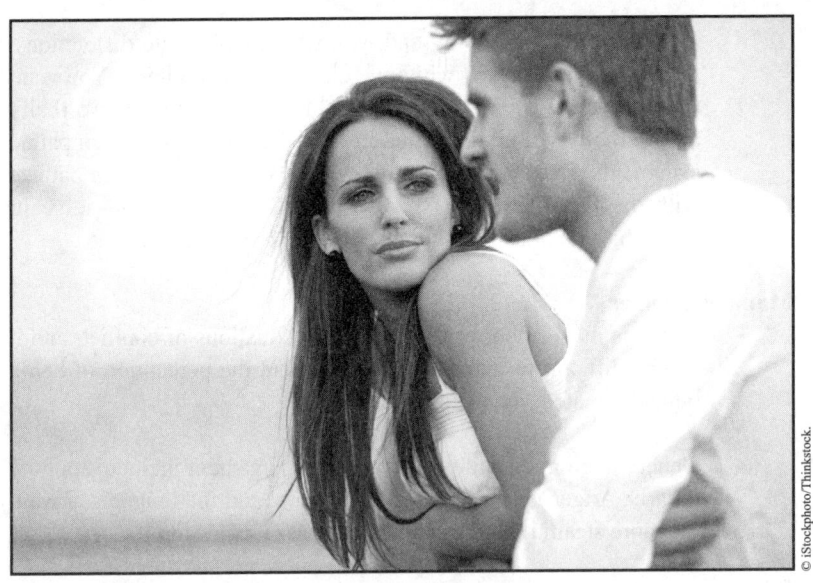

About half of all marriages end in divorce, and about 36 percent of Americans say that they're lonely.

- Men are also less likely to pick up on emotional cues and less likely to take turns or to give openings to other people. Essentially, when a man is talking to another person, he gives a report; on the other hand, women engage in rapport building.

- How can we improving our communication skills? Remember that there are two sides of the coin: sending and talking, and listening and receiving.

- For sending and talking, you need to pick a good time. An after-work ambush is not a good time to have a productive conversation. Know what you need, make it clear, and have realistic expectations. Just stick with one issue—no matter how many memories are activated because of your emotional state. Be aware of the verbal and nonverbal signals that you're sending to the other person.

- If you're on the receiving end, you want to eliminate distractions: Don't multitask or text while the other person is talking. You want to improve the signals that you send to your partner—nonverbally and verbally. Limit interruptions if possible, and use empathic statements. Even if you disagree with a person, you can empathize with the fact that he or she is upset. Don't rush in to solve it; sometimes he or she might just need you to listen first.

Managing Anger

- Anger is most often what comes up in situations of conflict, and it can be difficult to manage. Anger is about the perception of being unjustly treated, wronged, or cheated.

- General recommendations for anger management include stopping it early. Anger is like a fast-moving train, and the longer you wait, the more steam it picks up and the harder it is to stop it.

- Identify the trigger, or cause, of your anger. Ask yourself whether it's worth the investment of energy and resources; it costs your body a lot in terms of cardiovascular reactivity when you're angry.

- Strategies to help manage your anger include cognitive behavioral therapy and cognitive restructuring. Of course, you can challenge your habits of mind, such as personalization and magnification.

- Another strategy is to halt hostile fantasies. Often, we will have arguments in our mind with our spouse, even if they've never really occurred in reality.

- In addition, time-outs are not just for children; they're for adults, too. You need to make sure that both individuals in the couple are on board with the time-out and what that time-out means. It's not a free pass to withdraw; it's not a free pass for avoidance.

Suggested Reading

Beck, *Prisoners of Hate*.

Covey, *The 7 Habits of Highly Effective People*.

Gottman and Silver, *The 7 Principles for Making Marriage Work*.

Hendrix, *Getting the Love You Want*.

King and Straus, et al, *The Social Medicine Reader*.

McKay, Rogers, and McKay, *When Anger Hurts*.

Questions to Consider

1. What role does culture play in how intimacy and conflict are expressed or experienced? Are some cultures better at it than others?

2. What should you do in the case of an unsolvable conflict? Is it possible to "agree to disagree" without affecting intimacy?

Touched by Grace—Spirituality and Health
Lecture 19

This lecture focuses on spirituality and health. The challenge is to understand the meaning and purpose of religiosity and spirituality and how they relate to community and social support. In this lecture, you will learn about some of the attitudes and concepts that are held by many of the different world religions, including acceptance and forgiveness. In addition, you will be exposed to spirituality and health research, and you will begin to pull apart some of the mechanisms to expose what we know and what we don't yet know about this topic.

Spirituality and Health

- Spirituality is defined as the personal quest for understanding answers to ultimate questions about life, meaning, and relationships to the sacred or transcendent—which may or may not lead to or arise from the development of religious rituals in the formation of community.

- Religion is defined as an organized system of beliefs, practices, rituals, and symbols designed to facilitate closeness to the sacred or transcendent, God, higher power, some ultimate truth or reality—and to foster an understanding of one's relationship and responsibility to others living together in a community.

- Most people in the United States are more likely to consider themselves spiritual rather than religious. One of the predictors of positive emotion and health is religiosity. In fact, belonging to a religious community seems to have a stronger effect than simply being spiritual.

- There is a special relationship between spirituality, health, and illness because, although spirituality and religion is present at all times, when we are sick, we are especially challenged.

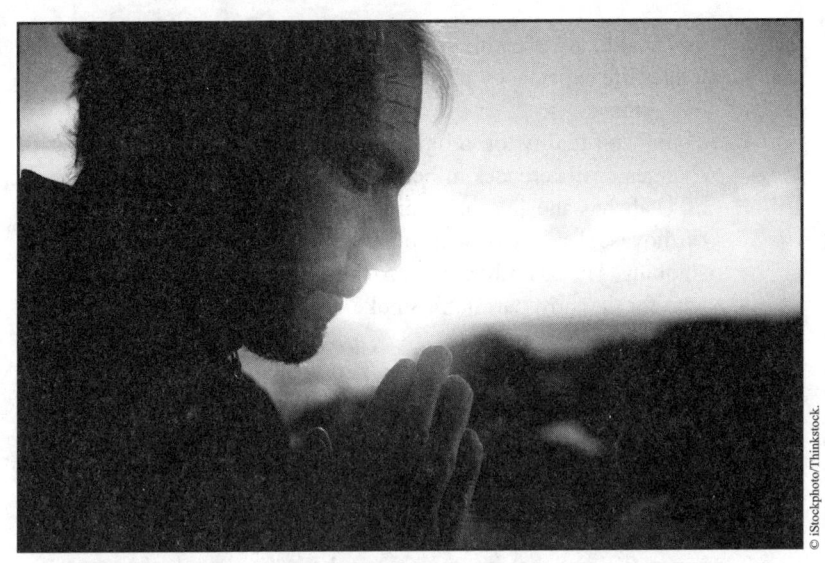

About 95 percent of Americans say that they believe in a higher power. About 90 percent say that they pray, while 70 percent say that they pray daily.

- For many people, religion or spirituality forms the basis of meaning and purpose in life. The profoundly disturbing effects of illness can call into question a person's purpose in life and work. Healing, the restoration of wholeness, as opposed to technically fixing someone, requires answers to these questions. Faith can be shaken or strengthened.

- In the early 20th century, William James thought that religion influenced our health—particularly through the central nervous system or the neurological system.

- Over subsequent decades, science became more focused on pragmatic, reductionistic research, and religion was essentially taboo. Studying religion was left to the theologians.

- In the past decade and a half, we've seen a great resurgence in the scientific understanding of what spirituality is and how it influences our health. In general, we've found lower overall mortality and longer life expectancy for religious or spiritual people.

- Could spirituality or religion and health be related because of changes or differences in health behaviors? For example, the state of Utah has the lowest smoking rate and, hence, lower rates of cardiovascular disease and other complications commonly due to smoking. This is probably due to the higher proportion of Mormons, who for the most part don't smoke, that live in Utah.

- In terms of social support, if you're part of an organized community, you're more likely to be getting regular in-person social support.

- In the cognition category, researchers talk about something called the sense of coherence, or sense of meaning. Having a religion or spirituality gives you a sense of meaning. Recall that the primary appraisals are what we think about the stressor while the secondary appraisal is about the resources.

- For people who believe in a higher power, there's always a resource and strategy. This may alter their primary, and most likely their secondary, appraisals. As a consequence, it may alter their stress response.

- Religion may foster solidarity and identity. We identify with a particular culture, and that often includes a set of spiritual or religious beliefs. Maybe religion assists people in giving up old objects of value and finding new sources of significance. We do some perspective shifting in what we think is important and what really matters.

- If we're talking about activating or deactivating our biological systems, there are two different categories of models. One is called direct effects. Maybe it's some neurobiological system that we just haven't discovered yet, or maybe it's the chemical oxytocin or vasopressin, which we really don't know much about yet.

- The second family of models is called stress-buffering effects. Maybe it's not a unique, different system that's helping us out. Maybe it's simply turning down the HPA axis or the sympathetic nervous system. Of course, these two models aren't mutually exclusive, so it could actually be both direct effects as well as stress-buffering effects.

Transcendental Meditation
- Interesting studies done in the area of blood pressure are primarily in the realm of meditation. The kind of meditation that is most studied is either mindfulness meditation or transcendental meditation. In many blood pressure studies, transcendental meditation has been used.

- Transcendental meditation is a meditation that relies on a mantra. In all of the different types of meditation, there's usually some level of somatic quieting. There's some kind of acceptance or developing a lack of judgment—developing positive regard.

- In transcendental meditation, there's also a focus on a mantra. Generally, people can write their own mantras, but with transcendental meditation, a spiritual guru writes your mantra for you.

- If you practice meditation daily, focusing on your mantra over and over, in a number of randomized control trials, systolic blood pressure drops by about 10 points, which is clinically significant in terms of improving your cardiovascular health. In addition, transcendental meditation and other forms of meditation may help lower overall cardiovascular reactivity, including blood pressure.

- The science of brain waves is fairly imprecise at this point, but we do know that when one particular type of brain wave—the gamma wave—is in synchrony, it looks like a smooth wave, and all of that noise has been erased. It's a measure of the quality of concentration.

- One of the key features of meditation is concentration. You concentrate on your breath, your mantra, or an image. When examining meditators, Richie Davidson at the University of Wisconsin found more gamma wave synchrony than they had ever seen in any population. All of that practice and training had made a difference in terms of their brain physiology.

- There are, of course, common practices across the different religions—including prayer, mantras, meditations, and rosaries—all of which perhaps have the same effects on our health.

- Some of the common attitudes across different religions that might be worth studying include acceptance, forgiveness, compassion, kindness, empathy, and altruism.

Ideas of Acceptance
- Ideas of acceptance are present in a number of different religions. Acceptance is the idea of having unconditional love—of not judging others. It is the idea of accepting that we're all inherently flawed humans and suffering is unavoidable.

- Many religions encourage us to cultivate an attitude of nonjudgment. They tell us, though, that acceptance is not resignation; it's a realization and appreciation of the inherent imperfections of life.

- Forgiveness is very much related to acceptance, and there's actually a number of scientific studies that have looked at the health effects of forgiveness. Many of these studies remind us that forgiveness is not about forgetting, surrender, resignation, or passivity.

- Forgiveness and reconciliation are different. Forgiveness is an active and ongoing process that might actually take years to evolve, and the primary beneficiary is the person doing the forgiving. The person who has wronged you may no longer be present. You're the one that benefits, particularly from a cardiovascular perspective.

- One of the best-known forgiveness studies, which came out of Stanford and was conducted by Fred Luskin and his colleagues, is called the Stanford forgiveness project. Through their research, they found that you can teach a person how to forgive, and they can get better at it.

- Predictors of forgiveness include the intent to forgive. It starts with a decision: the transgressor giving an apology, the capacity for empathy, and the ability to control anger. Situational factors—whatever the transgression might have been and the circumstances since then—are also fairly powerful.

- The path toward forgiveness starts with the decision to forgive, but it takes a while. Once you start to feel anger, you want to stop that fast-moving train. You want to try to switch tasks, or find a distraction. You want to do something to induce positive emotions.

- You also need to rewrite the story of what happened. That doesn't mean to fool yourself, but to try to take different perspectives, develop empathy skills, develop attributions, or change attributions. Remember that forgiveness is for you; it's not for someone else.

Suggested Reading

Chodron, *When Things Fall Apart*.

Dossey, *Prayer Is Good Medicine*.

Enright, *Forgiveness Is a Choice*.

King and Straus, et al, *The Social Medicine Reader*.

Koenig, King, and Carson, *Handbook of Religion and Health*.

Luskin, *Forgive for Good*.

Miller and Thoresen, "Spirituality, Religion, and Health."

Rosen, *Thank You for Being Such a Pain*.

Taylor, *My Stroke of Insight*.

Questions to Consider

1. If you were to perform a spiritual needs assessment on yourself, what would be your strengths? What are your areas of vulnerability? Can you recall a time in the past when your spiritual needs were not being met? What helped or hurt?

2. Is the value placed on forgiveness driven by a specific ideology, or does forgiveness have inherent value regardless of your belief system or cultural background? Why?

A Matter of Class—Socioeconomics and Health
Lecture 20

This lecture focuses on socioeconomic status and how it relates to health. The lecture will start by defining socioeconomic status (SES), which has three components: education, income, and social status. In this lecture, you will learn how SES is linked to health risks, health behaviors, the experience of stress, and overall rates of morbidity and mortality. You will learn that multiple pathways can be activated that help us understand the relationship between SES and health, including health care, physical environment, social environment, behavior, or stress.

Socioeconomic Status

- There are three components of socioeconomic status (SES): education, income, and occupational status. Education and income are correlated at about 0.4 (a perfect correlation would be 1.0 while a perfect negative correlation would be –1.0). Statistically, that means that education accounts for approximately 16 percent of the difference in income.

- This has to do with where you are on the educational trajectory. It is absolutely true that having a high school diploma versus not means that you'll make more money. It is also true, for the most part, that having a bachelor's degree versus not having one means that you're going to make more money. It's when you get into graduate school that it's a little different; some people will have lots of education but very little income.

- When we talk about SES and health, the threshold effects of poverty usually comes to mind. It's very easy to imagine a relationship between extreme poverty and health. The assumption is that once you have enough food, shelter, clothing, and decent insurance that you can access health care, then wealth shouldn't matter that much. This seems logical, but it isn't true.

- The first studies to demonstrate the fallacy of a poverty threshold were the Whitehall studies, Whitehall I and Whitehall II, led by Sir Michael Marmot in the United Kingdom. Their research showed that even after poverty is removed, earning more still improves your health, primarily measured in terms of life expectancy.

- As of 2011, per capita income in the United States is approximately $41,600. In Japan, per capita income is $32,000 while in China, it's $4,500. We're a wealthy country, and we have a lot of resources. However, the gap is widening.

- Education has improved in our country. More people are getting college degrees—both men and women, minority and nonminority. The United States lags a number of Asian countries in science and math test scores. We do have a number of high-status occupations.

- Given our SES, we do not have the best health. We are the sixth wealthiest in per capita income in the world. We're at number 34 in terms of infant mortality, and we're at number 38 in terms of life expectancy.

Components of SES: Income

- There is an unequivocal relationship between income and health: The more money you make, the better your health. The richest men and women in the United States could expect to live approximately 6.5 years longer. However, compared to international data on per capita income and longevity, rich Americans aren't living as long as they should.

- The link between income and health is related to access to health care. That doesn't mean that more expensive health care equals better health care, but sometimes that is the case.

- More income is linked to the ability to buy more nutritious food. In addition, income is related to being able to buy a home in a safe neighborhood and gives you access to exercise facilities. Income is related to the ability to pay for education.

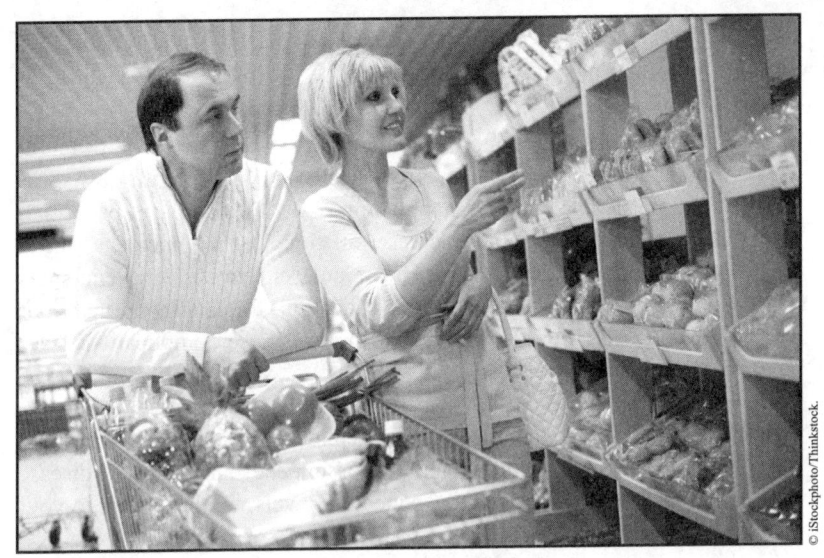

More income is linked to the ability to buy more nutritious food.

- If you have financial resources, it's going to alter your secondary appraisals. Altering secondary appraisals also alters your stress response—specifically, turning it down. You have less to worry about because you have more resources, less wear and tear on the system, and less allostatic load.

Components of SES: Education

- In terms of education, there have been dramatic improvements in subpopulations in the United States. For example, women now outnumber men in colleges. There has been greater diversification of high-status professions such as physicians, lawyers, and top-level executives. Still, the proportion of minorities in those professions nowhere matches their proportions in the general population.

- Those who have not finished high school are four times more likely to have poor health in general. On average, college graduates will live five years longer than high school dropouts. Children of high school dropouts are six times more likely to be in poor health compared to college graduates.

- Diabetes is increasingly common across a number of different populations, probably overrepresented in those with low SES and particular minority populations. Low education, in particular, is correlated with an increase in complication incidence rates among diabetics, including heart attacks, strokes, and end-stage renal disease. If you have low education, the likelihood that your diabetes is going to progress to one of those complications goes up dramatically.

- We can deduce that the link between income and education is about how our social circles facilitate or impede our efforts at disease management. Your friends' education levels will be similar to your own education level.

- Another variable that we think is at play is something called health literacy. Literacy in general is defined as an individual's ability to read, write, speak a language, and compute and solve problems using language or symbolic representations at levels of proficiency necessary to function on the job, in the family of the individual, and in society.

- Literacy is certainly related to education. Higher levels of education equal higher levels of literacy. The American Medical Association pushed this idea of literacy a little bit further. They wanted to look much more closely at this construct of health literacy, which is defined as the ability to obtain, process, and understand basic health information and services needed to make appropriate health decisions and follow instructions for treatment.

- Current data indicate that more than one-third of Americans, or about 89 million people, lack sufficient health literacy to effectively undertake and execute needed medical treatments and preventive health care.

- About 26 percent of Americans do not understand when their next appointment is scheduled. About 42 percent do not understand instructions to take medication on an empty stomach. Up to 78 percent misinterpret warnings on prescription labels, and 86 percent cannot understand the Rights and Responsibilities section of a Medicaid application.

- This is a failure both of our educational systems and medical system. We should be able to take care of people with a full range of abilities, literacies, health literacies, and languages. Of course, there's still responsibility on the side of the patient and family.

Components of SES: Occupational Status

- Occupational status is a little trickier than income and education. The status of professions changes over time. Sometimes entirely new professions emerge—for example, software engineer—and others disappear.

- Status is usually measured through questionnaires, in which there's a long list of different professions and people are asked to simply rank them. Usually in the top slots, we see physicians, engineers, superstar athletes, and firefighters. In the middle are teachers and bankers. In the lowest rungs, we see food preparation workers, bartenders, and janitors.

- The making of those subjective determinations of status is partly about training and education and about the complexity of the job. It's about the amount of income, but it's also about the power and influence that they have, as well as whatever cultural beliefs one might have about the value of that particular profession or what their contributions might be to society.

- The most common way that status is measured is with a very simple procedure developed by social psychologist Nancy Adler, who is interested in perception of status. As with social support, perception of status seems more important than the actual reality.

- Adler shows a simple picture of a ladder to an individual, who is instructed to place an X on the rung on which they believe they stand. There are two versions of the ladder: one linked to traditional SES indicators and the other linked to standing in one's community.

- The difference between these two ladders may be of particular interest in poorer communities where individuals may not be high in SES, but they may be high in terms of social reputation in their local or religious communities.

Questions about SES and Health

- Is it possible if your parents or grandparents were impoverished that they were epigenetically altered and that you inherit it? If you inherit it, can you change it? We don't quite yet have the answers to these questions.

- What about poverty in childhood? If you grew up in a poor family but were able to have a high-status profession, are you still damaged as a consequence of poverty in childhood? The answer is that it depends on how severe the deprivation was.

- Does wealth protect you in later life? As we get older, as our bodies slow down, the incidence of disease, mostly chronic diseases, gets much higher. If have had high SES as you go through young adulthood through middle age into older adulthood, is that like putting money in the bank, or is age the great leveler—regardless of your socioeconomic status? It depends on the disease, actually.

- In fact, for most chronic biological diseases, it is money in the bank. It slows down the progression of chronic disease or the likelihood that you might contract one. However, age is the great leveler for depression and other psychiatric illnesses. It seems that no matter how much money you have and how long you've had it, even rich people can get depressed.

Suggested Reading

Adler and Stewart, "Health Disparities across the Lifespan."

King and Straus, et al, *The Social Medicine Reader*.

Scott, "Life at the Top in America Isn't Just Better, It's Longer."

Questions to Consider

1. Given the importance of perceived social status (the "ladder"), would earned wealth and inherited wealth have the same positive impacts on health? Would they operate through the same mechanisms?

2. Could interventions to change people's perception of their socioeconomic status (e.g., by comparing themselves to global averages rather than U.S. averages) be sufficient to improve their health, even if their socioeconomic status doesn't objectively change? Should we do this if it works?

A Cog in the Wheel—Occupational Stress
Lecture 21

In this lecture, you will explore the concept of occupational, or work-related, stress. You will learn the definition of the concept, identify some key features, and look at both predictors as well as protective factors. You will also learn about some explicit links between occupational stress and the onset and exacerbation of disease. In addition, you will learn about chronic occupational stress, or burnout, and how to treat it. Hopefully, this lecture inspires you to think about your own workplace and changes that might help you experience less stress.

Occupational Stress

- About 30 percent of U.S. workers are often or always under a lot of stress at work. Measures of work stress have increased 300 percent since 1995. Problems at work are more strongly associated with health complaints than are any other types of stressors, including financial problems or family stressors.

- Occupational stress is stress that's caused by our work or occupations. That stress includes biological, emotional, behavioral, and cognitive components. Because we are humans, stressors don't have to actually be real or external in our environment. They can be about our interpretations, appraisals, or predictions, which happen in the workplace all the time.

- The top 10 most stressful occupations list is as follows.
    1. enlisted soldier in the military
    2. firefighter
    3. airline pilot
    4. air traffic controller

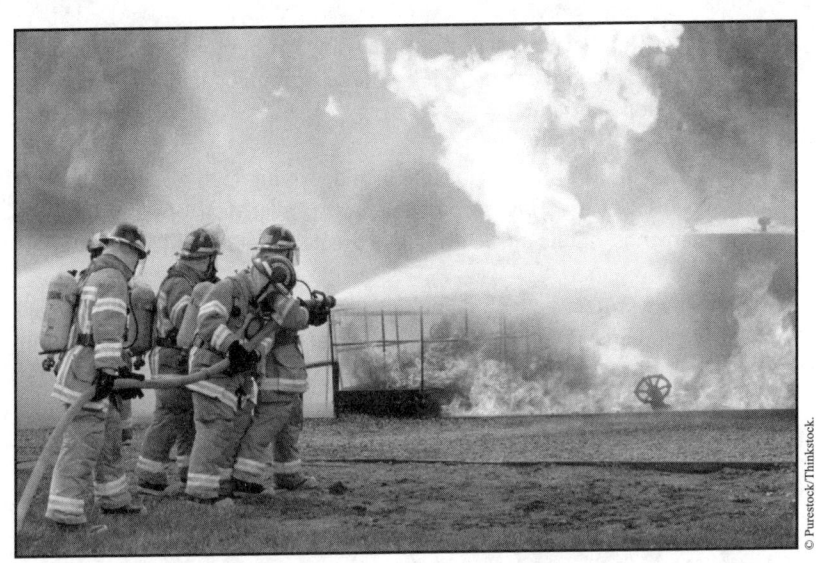

Surveys of occupational stress find that being a firefighter is the second most stressful occupation.

  5. police officer
  6. event coordinator
  7. inner-city school teacher
  8. taxi driver
  9. customer service operator
  10. emergency medical technician

- Some of the elements that those top 10 most stressful jobs have in common include work demands, work climate, perceived lack of control, and high demand or high job strain. It has to do with a great disparity between effort and reward. It also has to do with the individual perceiving the demands of his or her job as threats rather than as challenges.

- Occupational stress is the precursor for burnout. If it continues for long enough and if it is intense enough, then an individual develops burnout.

- Some of the protective factors include having high perceived control. The CEO of a big corporation has a great deal of stress and job demands, but he or she also has a great deal of reward and control.

- Other protective factors include having a high reward that matches high demand and having a high social status. It also has to do with having a sense of meaning or purpose.

- In 2000, Cox published some of his work in a book that helps us delineate the different factors in the workplace that contribute to stress. He these different factors into two categories: content and context.

- Content is not so much the task, or job, that you do; it's more about the circumstances of how you do it and some of the global characteristics. For example, are you working in a safe and supportive environment? What is the volume of work that you have to produce?

- Context is more about the work philosophy and the environmental conditions. For example, what are the goals of your particular job? What are the expectations of your employer? What is communication in the workplace like?

Measuring Occupational Stress
- To measure occupational stress, you must decide which level you'd like to focus on: Do you want to focus on the experience of the individual worker, a working group, or the overall workplace? Usually, the data gathered comes from a combination of self-report questionnaires, independent observers, and some amount of objective data.

- The usual measures of individual stress are similar to the perceived stress scale. The most commonly used is the occupational stress inventory, which contains 140 different items with three dimensions. It asks about occupational stress as well as psychological and emotional strain. It also addresses coping resources.

- A variant of this is the job stress survey, which contains only 30 items. It asks you to list the frequency and severity of different stressors. It takes a very different theoretical approach.

- The organizational climate questionnaire, which looks not at the individual but at the organization, contains 18 items that are divided into six dimensions. You answer on a 1-to-5 Likert scale, which ranges from "almost never" (1) to "very frequently" (5). The dimensions include organizational support, member quality, openness, supervisory style, member conflict, and member autonomy.

- The interesting thing about the organizational climate questionnaire is that you're making two ratings for each of the different items: an actual rating and an ideal rating. This gives us an idea of what you value and how close your actual environment is to your ideal work environment.

- Alternatively, you can assess your personal job tasks, content, and context by using some detailed self-monitoring, essentially creating a spreadsheet of different dimensions that you've deemed important and then recording what it is that you do throughout the course of three to five typical workdays, for example.

- You might also begin to dissect what it is about your particular job that provokes stress. For example, if you are asked to write a report and you feel incredibly stressed about it, you want to start digging in cognitive-behavioral fashion, asking yourself what it is about this particular assignment that is stressful—about the work task but also the context, expectations, and goals. Hopefully, you're also thinking about ways that you could address some of the problems you identify.

Medical Consequences of Occupational Stress

- What are some of the medical consequences of occupational stress? We're interested in it as a psychological phenomenon, but we also want to look at the effect it has on our bodies.

- The research has been divided into a number of different areas. The three most common are the relationship between work stress and cancer, work stress and back pain, and work stress and cardiovascular disease.

- There are no conclusive findings in regard to the relationship between work stress and cancer. There are studies that show that high levels of occupational stress are related to particular kinds of cancer, but it tends to be in professions where there are occupational exposures to carcinogens.

- People who have high occupational stress have up to three times the rate of back pain, and it's usually lower back pain. We believe that this is, in some part, due to the psychological experience of stress, but we don't yet understand the mechanisms.

- The strongest findings are in the realm of occupational stress and cardiovascular disease. The first comes from Kuper and was published in 2002. He found that a person who had high occupational stress had up to double the risk of having cardiovascular disease and of eventually having a heart attack.

- A similar study was done by Stephenson, but this one is unique in that it had a 25-year follow-up. Stephenson found that high job strain doubled the risk of death from heart disease and was associated with increased cholesterol and body mass index.

Burnout

- Burnout is related to stress, but it's more chronic. It's something that tends to build over time, and it isn't simply resolved by having a long weekend. When people are burned out, they're still working very hard, but they're less and less productive. They're becoming more negative, more cynical, and angrier. They have long-term exhaustion and less interest in their activities.

- The most common way to measure burnout is the Maslach burnout inventory, developed by Christina Maslach, a psychologist at the University of California, Berkeley. Maslach tells us that burnout has three different dimensions: emotional exhaustion, depersonalization, and cynicism. It's also about personal accomplishment—or accomplishing less and less over time.

- It is possible when a person is burned out that he or she might also meet criteria for a psychiatric disorder—specifically, something called an adjustment disorder, where a person experiences a stressful life event and become more impaired than one might usually predict. It might also be depression.

- There are some simple interventions that involve changing our workplace environments that can actually go a long way in terms of combating occupational stress and treating burnout. We can change things like the lighting, temperature, noise, and space. We need to decrease the ambiguity of the job and increase predictability.

- In companies where there is some level of shared decision making, where the employees have a voice, there tends to be less burnout and less occupational stress. There is also less burnout and stress when workers are given work assignments that are more interesting and variable, when social relationships at work are supported, and when rewards are given for good work over and above what an individual might have been expecting.

- Other ways to combat work stress include positive emotion exercises. You can keep a gratitude journal, which is perspective-shifting work. You can also use cognitive therapy skills, including positive reappraisals and wrestling with dysfunctional thoughts. You can work to recalibrate your perspectives and expectations.

- Usually, combating burnout requires an extended period of time away from work. It might require a change in job description. Individuals who are burned out potentially need a better work-life balance. They need time with family and friends rather than just time with coworkers or people that they might be serving in their job.

Suggested Reading

Cox, Griffiths, and Rial-Gonzalez, *Research on Work-Related Stress*.

King and Straus, et al, *The Social Medicine Reader*.

Maslach, *The Truth about Burnout*.

Questions to Consider

1. How do occupational stress and the stress of being unemployed compare? At what point would it be healthier to be unemployed rather than working in an unhealthy workplace?

2. Workers in the United States put in far more hours than many of their European counterparts. Could this difference partly account for the lower life expectancy in the United States? Are we literally working ourselves to death?

The Power of Place—Communities and Health
Lecture 22

This lecture uses the social-ecological model to help you understand how built-in social environments help answer the three questions of this course: Why do some people get sick? Why do other people stay well? What can we do about it? The social-ecological model isn't just about people and relationships or just about public health or health policies—that's the social part. The ecological part reminds us about the physical and structural environment around us and why it, too, matters.

Places: Communities and Neighborhoods

- Places can powerfully evoke emotions, and they can trigger those emotions—both good and bad. Triggered emotions trigger stress responses, good or bad. Certain places, such as your parents' home, are very powerful in being able to evoke memories and emotional states, which consequently affects our health.

- Places are related to identity—social in-groups, geography, neighborhood, county, and high school. Ecology influences our behavioral opportunities. Is it safe to go for a walk? Is healthy food available? It influences our choices; it's not just about willpower. Can we engineer environments that make us healthier?

- Let's look at some of the bigger divisions in terms of place—starting with the difference between urban and rural. The vast majority of Americans live in an urban setting, but historically that hasn't always been the case. Over the past century, we have seen a vast migration to urban settings. Different places mean different health consequences.

- There are also a number of different geographic distinctions in the United States, including the West Coast, the Deep South, the Midwest, and New England. There are different cultures and different health opportunities—risk factors as well as protective factors.

- How could we define community? Is it about the zip code? Is it a census tract? Is it about regulations? Is it about subcultures? Is it about self-identity? Communities are not just about spatial location. Some communities—for example, the Italian American community—might be spatially dispersed, but they consider themselves members of the same community.

- Some communities have a spatial relationship while others are more about social identity. Communities include behavioral opportunities and social supports. They also include stressors and environmental exposures and might have other negative health effects. Communities are also a resource, and they may show resilience.

- Neighborhoods are nested within a community, but they're also difficult to define. Researchers tend to agree that neighborhoods refer to a geographic unit of limited size with relative homogeneity in housing and population, as well as some level of interaction in symbolic significance to its residents. With this definition, neighborhoods change over time.

The Physical Environment

- There are two categories of features of an environment: physical features as well as social features. The physical environment includes how the land is used, the density of the population, and the type of housing that is available. This also includes transportation, street connectivity, schools, libraries, the food environment, and the recreational environment.

- The social environment includes having a sense of safety or violence, social cohesion or social capital, social norms, and collective efficacy. It also includes signs of disorder, or aesthetic quality.

- In terms of the physical environment, environmental exposures are the chemical or biological environment that's around us. A variety of health-related hazards are disproportionately found in low-income neighborhoods in housing, including excess moisture, mold, allergens, poor indoor air quality, structural deficiencies, and lead contamination.

- Occupational exposures to chemicals, physical overexertion or inactivity, excessive heat or cold, noise and psychosocial factors like stress or job strain can create or worsen a variety of health problems, including cancer, chronic obstructive pulmonary disease, asthma, and even heart disease.

- The food environment simply refers to the number, type, and distribution of food stores and food service establishments. Grocery stores, convenient stores, fast-food restaurants, and high-quality restaurants all fit into an individual's food environment.

- The available food within a mile or two of our homes, for example, can dramatically influence our food choices, especially in an urban area and especially for individuals that may not have ready access to transportation or to a car.

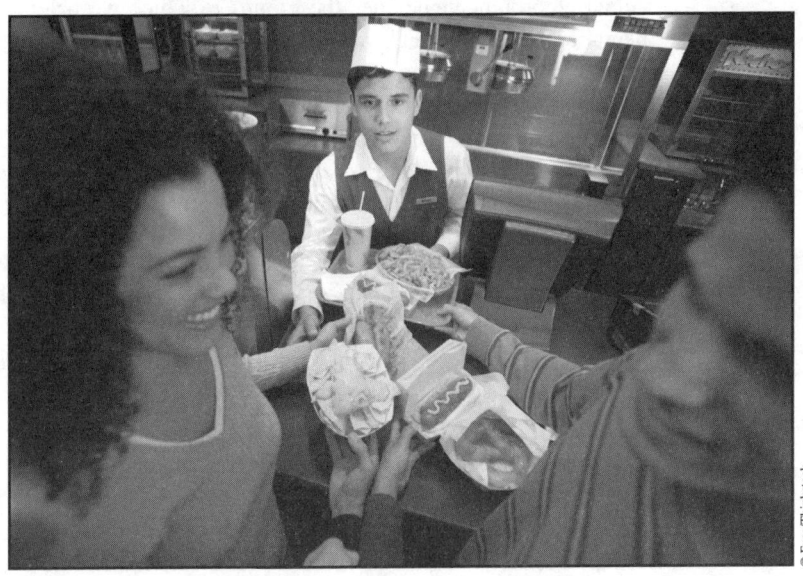

Having access to unhealthy food negatively affects health.

- Studies of children and adolescents have shown that the presence of convenience stores and fast-food restaurants is associated with a higher consumption of potato chips, chocolate, white bread, soda, and fast foods. Similarly, adults residing in a self-ranked poor food environment were significantly less likely to consume a healthy diet compared to adults who reside in a healthy food environment.

- We see a similar picture in the recreational environment. The research shows that access to recreational facilities, parks, sidewalks, bike lanes; the presence of neighborhood destinations such as shops or shopping areas and public squares; or having public transportation can lead to higher levels of physical activity.

- Conversely, higher crime rates and signs of physical disorder or decay may suggest an unsafe environment and will discourage individuals from being more physically active.

The Social Environment

- The social environment includes the groups to which we belong, the neighborhoods in which we live, the organization of our workplaces, and the policies that we create to order our lives. This includes social cohesion or social capital, collective efficacy, and the perception of safety or violence.

- Social capital is simply the time and energy invested in creating social bonds between individuals, or community members. It's about social networking and civic engagement. It's about personal recreation and other activities that create bonds between community members.

- Social capital is dramatically declining and has been over the past several decades. Research has shown that nearly all civic organizations have shown a marked decrease in enrollment and participation.

- Collective efficacy is defined as social cohesion among neighbors, combined with their willingness to intervene on behalf of the common good. This is a belief that by working together, the community can accomplish something.

- High collective efficacy is correlated with lower crime, higher community satisfaction, and higher safety in a neighborhood.

- Neighborhood safety includes physical decay, gangs, crime, and fast motor vehicle traffic. Physical decay, in a sense, tells criminals that people in the neighborhood don't care, so they're easy targets.

- Social epidemiologist Irene Yen tells us that to improve diet quality and physical activity, physicians need to get clever. She has recommended things like issuing vouchers for fruits and vegetables and establishing incentives for farmers' markets at community-based hospitals. Physicians should prescribe neighborhood park use and provide walking maps for the patient's neighborhood.

- We should also be looking at partnerships with community organizations. At San Francisco General Hospital, there is a group called Heart Beets that has two programs to promote healthy eating for low-income patients. It's not just about the government doing something; it's about the communities doing something for one another.

- We have our neighborhood health centers, which are, of course, involved in education and promotion of health. We are looking now at telemedicine, of ways to reach people in distant areas to improve their quality of health care. We're looking at interventions to improve community cohesion and involvement.

Changing Our Built Environment

- How can we change our built environment to be healthier? There are four different aspects of the built environment: contact with nature, buildings, public spaces, and urban form. Public spaces, for example, can be reengineered so that there are green spaces, walking trails, bike trails, and easily accessible public transportation.

- In terms of the natural environment, also called biophilia, we know that contact with nature has been associated with a number of interesting health outcomes, including fewer sick call visits among prisons, improved attention from children with attention deficit disorder, improved self-discipline among inner-city girls, decreased mortality among senior citizens, lower blood pressure and anxiety for people who have dental problems, and better pain control for bronchoscopy patients. Exposure to the natural environment reduces stress and enhances work performance.

- The second part of the built environment is about buildings. We have what are called sick buildings or healthy buildings, which involves an assessment of the quality of the air or of the temperature and the building materials that were used. In addition, is there easy access to healthy food, and is there appropriate lighting in order for people to do their jobs?

- The third part of the built environment is public places, which includes things like streets, sidewalks, and traffic flow. Is it safe to walk around? Is there appropriate lighting at night? Are there events, buildings, and places that promote social interactions or physical activities, parks, or public natural spaces?

- The fourth part of the urban environment is the urban form, which arises from the design, such as transportation and land-use decisions that have happened on a larger, usually governmental, scale. This influences whether or not people will migrate to suburbs and the commuting corridors in how long it takes people to commute. This is also where zoning codes come from.

Suggested Reading

Bronfenbrenner, *The Ecology of Human Development*.

King and Straus, et al, *The Social Medicine Reader*.

Ulrich, "View through a Window May Influence Recovery from Surgery."

Questions to Consider

1. Membership in a community can sometimes be more a matter of identity than geography—for example, belonging to the Jewish community. Do we select which communities we will belong to, or do they choose us? If we belong to more than one community, which one exerts the strongest affect on health?

2. How can we create healthy neighborhoods in densely populated urban areas? Conversely, how can people in sparsely populated rural areas feel connected to one another?

The Master Plan—Public Health and Policy
Lecture 23

This lecture explores the realm of public health. In this lecture, you will learn how to define public health. You will be given a broad overview and some basic examples of public health initiatives. In addition, this lecture will introduce you to a particular toolbox, a set of interventions, that is increasingly being used by public health officials: behavioral economics and choice architecture. You will learn about how these concepts push us to make bad choices, but also how we might use them to our advantage and be supported in making healthier choices.

Public Health
- Public health is the science and art of preventing disease, prolonging life, and promoting health through the organized efforts and informed choices of society, public and private organizations, communities, and individuals. Public health is about fulfilling society's interest in assuring conditions in which people can be healthy.

- Public health has essentially shifted its primary focus of battling epidemics of acute infectious diseases to tackling chronic diseases and, more recently, to helping us prepare for possible threats to community health, such as bioterrorism or new diseases like HIV/AIDS, SARS, or H1N1.

- The primary tasks of public health include the prevention of disease and injury; the promotion of health and well-being; the assurance of conditions in which people can be healthy; and the provision of timely, effective, and coordinated health care.

- The primary actors in the public health system include the community, the health-care delivery system, and our employers and businesses. It includes the media, academia, and government and the public health infrastructure.

- In today's public health world, we have a rather vast and complex system of private and public agencies, domestic and international, who share the common goals of improving our health.

- These include federal and local agencies, such as the Centers for Disease Control, the Food and Drug Administration, state health departments, and county health officials, but it also includes health educators, social workers, public health nurses, nonprofit agencies, and even the sanitation workers in your local neighborhood. One of the biggest challenges in public health today is how to direct this veritable orchestra of different players.

- Public health departments do many things for us, including monitoring health status to identify any emerging problems and informing, empowering, and educating people about health. They also help to mobilize community partnerships to solve health problems. Public health organizations help to enforce laws and regulations for public safety, research social factors relevant to health, and develop new interventions to improve health.

- Some of the success stories of public health include vaccinations, seatbelts, safe and clean drinking water, family planning, reductions in tobacco use, safer workplaces, prenatal medical care, and care and education for toddlers and preschoolers.

- Public health aims to prevent and treat disease, but it also seeks to improve health more broadly—to improve environmental or contextual factors that influence health—and it wants to help engineer a health-care system to meet the needs of the public. Given this breadth and our rather limited resources, there has to be a set of goals or guiding principles.

- In the service of developing this vision, the Department of Health and Human Services, a federal agency, developed a systematic approach to promoting health of the public in 1979. They called it the Healthy People initiative and decided that every 10 years, they

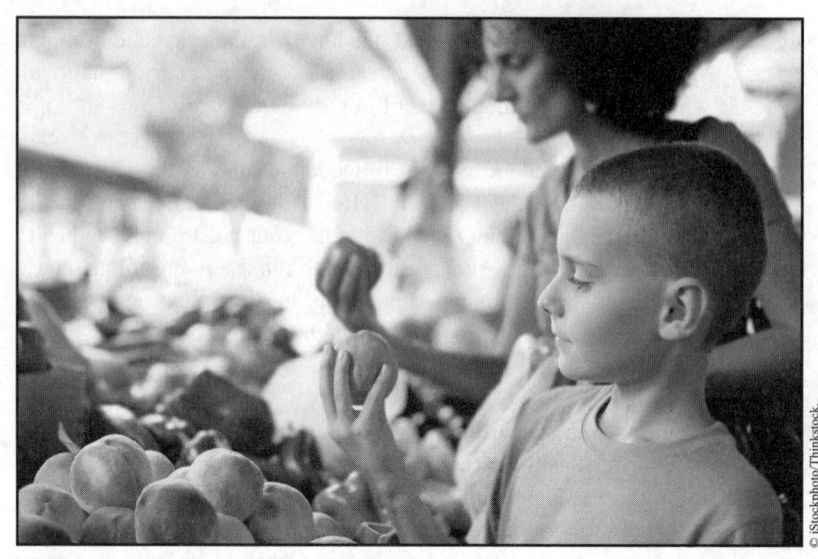

In some states, healthy foods do not have a sales tax, while junk foods do.

would have a different set of goals that all public health officials would work toward.

- Healthy People 2010 focused on two overarching goals: to increase the quality of life (including years of healthy life) and to eliminate health disparities (differences in both the onset of disease as well as the outcome of disease in different populations).

- In terms of the first goal, life expectancy has increased a few percent. Unfortunately, in terms of the second goal, health disparities have actually gotten worse—or we've gotten better at detecting, measuring, and publicizing those health disparities. Either way, we know that health disparities still exist.

- In Healthy People 2020, there are four overarching goals. There is still the goal about the quality of life, but the quantity has been nudged up. They want to dig a little deeper and figure out how to measure and improve quality of life for all Americans. They're interested in healthy development, so they're looking at children and their development into adulthood. They want to promote healthy behaviors across the entire life span. They want to look at social and physical environments that promote health.

- In Healthy People 2020, there are 42 topic areas, 600 objectives, and 1,200 measures. Fortunately, they have pulled out 26 leading health indicators that are only in 12 topics.

Behavioral Economics

- Behavioral economics seeks to unite the basic principles of classic economics with the realities of human psychology; in other words, it looks at how people are predictably irrational.

- As human beings, we are not particularly good at logical information processing. We make errors all the time, and we have all sorts of biases. We use what are called cognitive heuristics, or thinking shortcuts, as a way to conserve our computing energy.

- We do things like underestimate the likelihood that we will get a disease. We overestimate the likelihood of a reward or of positive things happening to us in the future. We have a known, and difficult to change, bias of preferring immediate gains; we don't care so much about punishments that come at some point down the road.

- Traditional economics talks about people who are often rational choosing to maximize their gain and minimize their losses. In utility theory, an economist would essentially write out an equation that would represent a social decision. He or she would consider benefits to you and to society. Using an equation, the economist would discover the choice that a rational person should make.

- We've learned that people don't actually make decisions that way. Instead, people make unhealthy choices. We're rather easily swayed by marketing and advertising that pushes us to make unhealthy choices.

- Behavioral economists, especially those of the public health persuasion, are trying to exploit these human tendencies to our favor. We're constantly being bombarded with marketing and carefully structured retail messages that push us to do something that we normally wouldn't have chosen.

- We can actually use behavioral economics to influence us to make healthier choices. We can educate consumers against the manipulations, which are most likely not going to stop, but we can also engineer systems that influence us to make better choices.

- There have been a number of public policy triumphs that fall within the realm of behavioral economics. For example, since the 1960s, smoking rates have dropped to just below 20 percent. One intervention was the increase in cigarette taxes. There is a direct relationship between the amount of cigarette tax and how many people choose to smoke. States that have the highest cigarette taxes have the fewest smokers, and vice versa.

Choice Architecture

- Choice architecture is about designing a system that influences our choices to go a particular way. It doesn't necessarily have to be about health; it might involve changing driving or shopping behavior.

- There are many possibilities for choice architecture. This could include the placement or appearance of stairs in public buildings to encourage people to take the stairs instead of elevators. This might also include incentivizing farmers' markets and putting them in places where people actually need them. This might involve building sidewalks, green spaces, and parks.

- There are different online sites that try to help people motivate behavior. These sites use behavioral economics to try to influence you to think more about long-term consequences and to also experience rewards or punishments upfront.

- For example, on a website called stickK.com, you set your own goals and identify a referee that will report whether you're sticking with your goal. In terms of smoking, the idea is that the benefit of smoking is upfront whereas the punishment is down the road. This website brings the punishment upfront so that the benefit of smoking is beside the punishment of smoking.

- On stickK.com, you enter your credit card number and specify an amount that you will pay if you cheat—if you smoke a cigarette, for example. That payment goes to what they call an anti-charity, someone that you would never want to give money to. If you smoke, your credit card is going to start paying that anti-charity. The punishment is memorable and proximal.

- The big debate is whether we should use carrots or sticks—rewards or punishments. Of course, either is going to work. People have argued that punishments are actually a little fairer and more economical. If you're using a reward for anyone that eats healthy, you're rewarding people who are doing it for the reward but people who would have done it anyway. That's a wasted reward from an economic standpoint.

Suggested Reading

Ariely, *Predictably Irrational*.

King and Straus, et al, *The Social Medicine Reader*.

Thaler and Sunstein, *Nudge*.

Questions to Consider

1. Given the nearly unavoidable presence of choice architecture in our daily lives, how can we inoculate ourselves against those influences and make more intentional, rational choices?

2. What do you see as the biggest public health challenges of the present? What successes or failures can you recall from your lifetime that might help shape our future interventions?

Heart and Soul—Cardiovascular Disease I
Lecture 24

In this lecture, you will learn about the anatomy, physiology, and pathophysiology of our cardiovascular system, focusing on myocardial infarction. You will learn about acute stress and cardiovascular changes, especially in vulnerable individuals. You will also learn about type A personality and, especially, hostility. This lecture will also examine a new type of research on type D personality. In addition, you will learn that depression has a fairly strong link to onset, progression, and recurrence of cardiovascular disease.

The Cardiovascular System and Cardiovascular Diseases

- The cardiovascular system is like plumbing, with the heart as the pump and the circulatory system as the pipes. The circulatory system is made up of primarily three different groups: arteries, veins, and capillaries.

- Arteries are dynamic and responsive, meaning that they can change their diameter. They can vasodilate to get larger and vasoconstrict to get smaller. Veins are tubes that bring deoxygenated blood and waste back to our hearts. Capillaries get so small that the epithelium, the lining of the capillaries themselves, are just one cell thick.

- Our circulatory system carries energy, oxygen, and nutrients to tissues, and it carries waste away. This is all done with our blood, which is made up of plasma (the watery, clear part of blood that accounts for 55 percent of blood), red blood cells (which contain hemoglobin in their cytoplasm), and white blood cells.

- The family of cardiovascular diseases is quite large. The top cause of hospitalization for adults over the age of 65 is congestive heart failure, which occurs because the heart is just not able to work hard enough to pump the blood as much as it needs to.

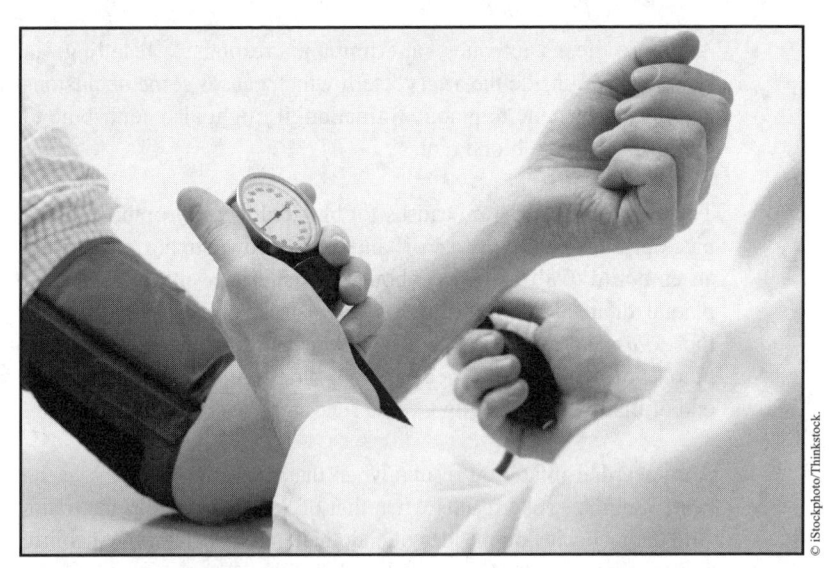

Hypertension, also known as high blood pressure, causes damage to blood vessels, tissues, and organs over time.

- Other diseases include cardiomyopathy, which is a disease of the heart muscle itself. In addition, there are peripheral vascular disease, aneurysms, and stroke.

- Myocardial infarctions are heart attacks. Arteriosclerosis refers to the loss of elasticity of the arteries, or the hardening of the arteries. It is a broad category that can mean a number of different things. Atherosclerosis, a narrowing of the arteries, is a kind of arteriosclerosis that is characterized by the deposition of lipids or fats and other blood-borne material within the arterial wall.

- Hypertension, or high blood pressure, over time causes damage to our blood vessels as well as to our tissues and organs. We believe this occurs through the shear stress model, which tells us that over a period of time, high blood pressure causes micro tears to occur inside the blood vessels.

- A micro tear activates an immune response, resulting in inflammation inside the artery itself, which causes some occlusions and may contribute to plaque formation. It might also contribute to the formation of a blood clot.

- There are many different causes for blood clots or thrombi. When a piece of a thrombus breaks off and moves downstream, it is called an embolus. We're worried about this material—either a ruptured plaque or an embolus—moving downstream because eventually, those vessels get smaller and smaller, resulting in occlusion and blood not being able to get past that blockage. Whatever's on the end of that pathway is going to be starved.

- A myocardial infarction results when that starvation happens in the heart itself. A stroke results when that occlusion occurs in the brain. Add to that occlusion the idea of endothelial dysfunction, the inability to dilate or to constrict as needed, and that's the equation that helps us understand why cardiovascular problems are so serious.

Stroke

- The pathophysiology of strokes is in some ways similar to that of myocardial infarctions. There are actually two common kinds of strokes. The first, which is more common, is called an ischemic stroke. It is similar to a myocardial infarction, but it essentially occurs in the brain.

- With an ischemic stroke, there's some sort of cutoff of blood supply, oxygen, and nutrients to the brain, and the brain tissues actually starve. Approximately 87 percent of all strokes are ischemic strokes.

- The other kind of stroke, which is much less common, is a hemorrhagic stroke. Instead of an occlusion, there is actually a weakened blood vessel that ruptures. An aneurysm is a common type.

- A transient ischemic attack is a ministroke, or a warning stroke. It may only last for a few minutes, and it has no lasting damage, but it tells you that something is not right and that you probably need a workup. With stroke, our carotid arteries in the sides of our neck are often key, but smaller vessels can be important as well, and all of them need to be checked out.

- With both myocardial infarctions and stroke, we need to think about prevention, treatment, and rehabilitation.

- Where does stress fit in? Many things happen when people are stressed, especially in their stress-response systems. Stress is normal, and the impact on our cardiovascular system is normal: The system gets ramped up, and then it comes back down. That is the cycle with normal stressors of daily life. We're most interested in individuals who have preexisting disease.

- Cardiovascular reactivity is mediated by the sympathetic nervous system. When you have a fight-or-flight response, you want some sort of activation. There is variability between individuals.

- Some of us have a very sensitive trigger while others have a very insensitive trigger. Some of us have a very high, or intense, cardiovascular response while others have a more modest response. Some of us have a response that is very long in duration while others have a much shorter response. Sensitivity, intensity, and duration of cardiovascular reactivity are all important in understanding why one person has a heart attack while another does not.

Cardiovascular Reactivity: Innate or Learned?
- Is our cardiovascular reactivity innate or learned? There is probably a genetic component, but there might also be a learned component based on some interesting epidemiologic findings.

- In general, cardiovascular reactivity is higher in men—in particular, it is higher in men who score high on scales of hostility. It is also higher in people who have grown up in impoverished environments, who have low socioeconomic status. Their cardiovascular systems were essentially trained that they need to have a robust and long-lasting response to deal with a hostile world.

- Another variable is heart rate variability. You want high heart rate variability. If you think of it in terms of flexibility, it means that you can quickly respond and quickly come back down, with minimal cost to the individual.

- Heart rate variability can be measured by looking at an electrocardiogram and taking the standard deviation of normal to normal heart beats. This gives you an idea of how flexible your system is and how well your parasympathetic nervous system is working.

- It looks like we might be able to improve heart rate variability with exercise, social support, and meditation. Some current research involves trials where they're looking at antidepressants to see if that might improve heart rate variability.

Type A, Type D, and Depression

- Type A personality style is a behavioral and emotional style marked by an aggressive, unceasing struggle to achieve more and more in less time, often in competition with other individuals or forces. There are three key elements: easily aroused hostility, time urgency, and competitiveness.

- There have been a number of dismantling studies that have tried to pull apart those three elements to see which one of those is actively contributing to cardiovascular disease and heart attack. If are very time urgent, you can relax. If you're competitive, you can relax—unless you have hostility that goes along with your competitiveness. It's really about easily aroused hostility.

- There are many studies that link hostility with cardiovascular disease. We often measure hostility with a questionnaire. For example, on the Cook-Medley hostility scale, we're worried about people who score in the top 20 percent.

- Type D personality style (where the "D" stands for "distressed") is a personality style that is receiving a lot of attention and seems to be related to cardiovascular disease. Someone who is type D has a lot of negative affect, such as anxiety, worry, sadness, and depression. This is a neurotic individual who is also socially inhibited and tends not to turn to his or her social supports.

- Shockingly, the prevalence of type D personality is estimated at 20 to 35 percent of the population. If a person scores high on a type D scale, he or she has a worse prognosis after having a heart attack—specifically, four to eight times the risk of having a second heart attack.

- Clinical depression is considered a medical disorder. It's not everyday blues or ups and downs. In fact, you have to have five out of nine symptoms that are present most of the day, nearly every day, for at least two weeks. These symptoms include having a low mood; not being able to enjoy things; having changes in appetite, weight, sleep, concentration, or memory; feeling worthless or guilty; or even having thoughts about suicide.

- There is a vast literature linking depression with cardiovascular outcomes. Essentially, if an individual is depressed, he or she is more likely to have a heart attack or cardiac events and less likely to recover after something happens.

Suggested Reading

Martz and Livneh, *Coping with Chronic Illness and Disability*.

Satterfield, *Minding the Body*.

Questions to Consider

1. Why do men tend to have higher cardiovascular reactivity than women? What advantages might this confer?

2. Which mechanisms might explain the link between type D personality and survival after a heart attack? Which interventions might help improve outcomes for this population?

Heart and Soul—Cardiovascular Disease II
Lecture 25

This lecture focuses on the biopsychosocial interventions to prevent or treat cardiovascular disease. In this lecture, you will learn what is based on evidence, what is promising but maybe yet unproven, and what is simply just not that effective. In addition to learning about changing behaviors, you will learn some general stress management interventions and whether they help cardiovascular outcomes. You will also look a little more generically at anger management interventions. Finally, you will examine the treatment of depression in relation to cardiovascular outcomes. You will discover that high-quality treatments for cardiovascular disease should be multimodal.

Types of Interventions for Cardiovascular Disease

- Behavior change intervention for cardiovascular disease includes things like smoking cessation, diet, exercise, and medical adherence. We typically think about these in terms of prevention, but they continue to be important even after disease onset. In that case, we want to slow disease progression and prevent future cardiovascular events from occurring.

- Over the past 35 years, the U.S. age-adjusted mortality from cardiovascular disease has declined by about 50 percent. This includes advances in diagnosis, prevention, and treatment (biomedical, behavioral, and psychological treatment).

- These gains are attributable to a wide menu of different options—including advances in medications, angioplasties, and stents—but it's also about lifestyle modifications and, particularly, about changes in smoking.

- If two smokers have a heart attack, but one stops smoking and the other continues, the one who stopped smoking will see a 36 percent reduction in mortality. This is by far the most important behavioral intervention that anyone can undertake.

- Within the first 24 hours of quitting smoking, smokers' circulation improves. They have less carbon monoxide in their system, and their red blood cells are better able to carry oxygen.

- In fact, half of the excess risk of cardiovascular disease goes away in the first 24 hours. The second half of that excess risk goes away within three years. This means that if a person stops smoking, within three years, his or her risk of having a heart attack goes back to the normal level of risk that we see in someone who hasn't ever smoked.

- Of course, this isn't true for cancer. About half of the risk of having cancer in a smoker goes away within 10 years, but we're not sure if the other half ever goes away. It's possible that the likelihood to have mutagenesis and cancers remains for the remainder of the individual's life.

- What about diet and nutrition? The American Heart Associate recommends dietary counseling as the cornerstone of coronary heart disease management. They've been extremely successful in educating the public.

- We know that we are supposed to limit our intake of saturated and trans fats. In addition, we're supposed to limit our intake of cholesterol and calories. We're supposed to lower or manage our weight if we need to. We should eat more whole grains, nuts, legumes, fruits, vegetables, and olive oils. Does the research support this?

- The seminal work of Dean Ornish showed us that not only can we slow cardiovascular disease, but we can actually reverse cardiovascular disease even in moderate or severe cases, just by using lifestyle interventions such as having a low-fat diet, becoming vegetarian, managing stress, and having regular and pretty intensive exercise.

- Medication interventions can essentially affect every piece of cardiovascular physiology. There are drugs that affect blood pressure, heart function, vasodilation, and blood thinning or clotting. We're also starting to see a pharmacotherapy movement that involves using some of those drugs to change psychological variables, including treating depression and psychiatric disorders but also hostility.

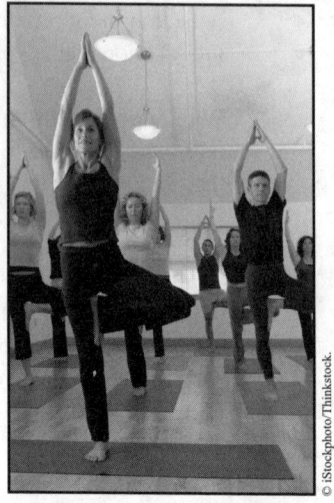

Exercise, such as yoga, helps with the management of stress.

Stress and Anger Management

- There is a menu of options that we have available to decrease an individual's experience of stress. Recall that cognitive behavioral therapy involves a triangle made up of thoughts, emotions, and behaviors, and all of those elements are interdependent. If you want to change the way a person feels, you might change his or her thoughts or behaviors, for example.

- When an individual experiences a stressor, it's not the stressor that makes him or her feel a certain way—it's the way he or she appraises the stressor, which is a form of cognition that we can work on to change.

- We want to learn ways to challenge our thoughts and to more effectively use our social supports. There's a family of behavioral interventions that includes exercise, relaxation, and somatic quieting, which involves changing our balance of activities—spending more time with family or friends, for example—so that we are doing more of what we want to instead of what we have to and doing things that give us a sense of both mastery and pleasure.

- A meta-analysis, or a summary of a number of different studies, was published by Wolfgang Linden in the *European Heart Journal* in 2007. It is a summary of 43 different randomized, controlled trials that were done. In these trials, they looked at psychological treatment compared to treatment as usual.

- They found that psychological treatment reduced cardiac patient mortality by 27 percent over follow-ups of two years or less. Event recurrence dropped to 43 percent when the follow-up was longer than two years. They also found, though, that the psychological treatment needed to be initiated at least two months after the cardiac event in order to produce the greatest benefit. They learned, too, that women with cardiac disease did not benefit as much as men.

- Recall the linkages between hostility and cardiovascular disease. It's a different question to show that hostility contributes to cardiovascular disease than to show that treating hostility improves cardiovascular disease. It might not be a two-way street.

- What are the interventions that we can teach to an individual that might have a problem with anger? This is the category of anger management.

- Some of the things that we want to do involve general cognitive behavior therapy skills. Recall that all of our emotions are there for a reason; they have a particular function or purpose. Each of the different emotions has a particular theme, or constellation of cognitions, that tends to go with them.

- When individuals are angry, they tend to have thoughts about some sort of violation or injustice that has occurred. Someone has taken something from them that was rightfully theirs or somehow harmed or insulted them. When you think about anger in angry cognitions—when you want to wrestle with those cognitions and do some cognitive restructuring—they're usually of that particular flavor.

- For people who have very quick tempers or tend to be angry a lot, they tend to overpersonalize. When something happens to them, they assume that it was intentional and targeted directly at them. They also tend to magnify, making mountains out of molehills, where something that was maybe just a slight accidental infraction becomes personal and a very big deal.

- The other thing that happens with anger is that individuals have a way of feeding that anger. Once it starts picking up steam, it's very difficult to stop.

- In fact, as human beings, we can make ourselves angry even when no one else is around and really nothing has happened. We're just imagining a past argument, or we might be imagining a future confrontation that hasn't even happened yet. We're coming up with good zingers; we're deciding what we're going to say. We're also increasing cardiovascular reactivity.

- One intervention of anger management strategies is to halt those hostile fantasies—to stop angry rumination. Interventions include things that we normally think of for children, including time-outs and cooling-off periods. These strategies are important for individuals, but they are certainly important for adult couples as well.

- We want to look at the use of alcohol or any other judgment-impairing things that people might do that involve losing control of their anger. We want to see if maybe the anger is just a surface manifestation of pain, depression, or fatigue or if it is maybe a result of other medical problems that an individual might be having. If so, of course, we want to treat those other problems.

- What about the research? The short answer is that we don't have much research yet that shows that anger management improves cardiovascular outcomes. The impact of anger management strategies on coronary heart disease is sort of a hot area right now, but we don't quite have the answers yet.

- From a number of meta-analyses, we do know that cognitive behavioral therapy works to reduce anger. In fact, it works quite well. We're just not sure if this reduction in anger translates into cardiovascular gains or not.

Treating Depression

- What about depression? Does treating the depression change cardiovascular outcomes? For cardiac psychologists and cardiologists who are interested in depression, it has been sort of the Holy Grail to show that you can treat depression and improve cardiovascular outcomes. Unfortunately, the search continues.

- Even though we know without a question that depression worsens cardiovascular outcomes, we do not yet know that treating depression improves cardiovascular outcomes. There may be a relationship, but we're not quite sure.

- It might be about health-related behaviors, but there haven't been any studies that have looked at health-related behaviors just yet. Maybe if we reach in and directly try to change the behaviors, we might see a difference.

Suggested Reading

Bath, Bohin, Jone, and Scarle, *Cardiac Rehabilitation*.

Kabat-Zinn, *Full Catastrophe Living*.

Martz and Livneh, *Coping with Chronic Illness and Disability*.

Satterfield, *Minding the Body*.

Questions to Consider

1. If your primary and secondary appraisals are balanced and fair, what good is cognitive therapy in helping you cope with a very real and possibly unchangeable stressor?

2. How can you use what you have learned from the earlier behavior change lectures to motivate yourself to stick with a meditation program? Be sure to use motivational interviewing techniques on yourself.

The Big C—Cancer and Mind-Body Medicine
Lecture 26

In this lecture, you will review cancer basics, especially factors that contribute to the onset and progression of cancer. You will also examine treatments, particularly those that involve stress and social support. You will discover whether biopsychosocial interventions have a role in the treatment of cancer. This lecture should leave you with a sense of hope and direction for where we need to go in the future to improve both our understanding of what causes cancer and the best ways to treat cancer—as well as the best ways to support patients and families.

Cancer Basics
- Cancer is a large family of diseases whose one common feature is an aberration in normal cell reproduction and regulation. Mutations occur during cellular reproduction, and if conditions are just right and the cells are not destroyed by the immune system, these mutated cancer cells rapidly reproduce, despite restrictions of space, nutrients shared by other cells, or signals sent from the body to stop reproduction.

- Mutations occur from a process called mutagenesis, in which genetic material is accidentally changed from a DNA copying error, for example, resulting in a mutation. These accidents may be spontaneous, or they may be caused by a mutagen, for example, being exposed to radiation or some sort of chemical toxin.

- Mutations can create diseases like cancer, but they're also considered to be the driving force behind traditional evolution. Of course, we have a number of natural safeguards to protect us from mutations, including oncogenes, tumor suppressor genes, and mismatch repair genes, which all help regulate the normal growth of cells.

- When cancer occurs, the on/off switch for oncogenes genes is somehow turned off. Tumor suppressor genes recognize abnormal growth and interrupt reproduction until a correction can occur, essentially applying the brakes on the process. Mismatch repair genes help us to recognize errors when DNA is copied to make a new cell and correct the error.

- Unfortunately, for many of us, eventually all three of these safeguards will fail. Tumors are an abnormal growth of tissue or a cluster of cells that are capable of growing and dividing uncontrollably. The normal processes of cellular regulation essentially fail.

- As these tumors grow, they consume resources and even stimulate the growth of new blood vessels to feed themselves in a process called angiogenesis. Without angiogenesis, tumors can't grow—they starve to death—so an entirely new line of treatments using angiogenesis inhibitors has been developed.

- As tumors grow, they might also metastasize, or send cancer cells into the bloodstream that might then take root, in a sense, in other parts of the body.

- Cancer cells are often shaped differently from healthy cells, and they don't function properly. Space and nutritional limitations don't seem to stop their growth. They just keep growing. They infiltrate, crowd, compress, and starve out normal tissues. The term "cancer" is used when a tumor is malignant, which means that it has the potential to cause harm, including death.

- Cancers are either detected with regular screening tests, such as the PSA screening for prostate cancer, or through imaging, such as mammograms for breast cancer. A workup, though, might be triggered by unexplained physical symptoms like fatigue, weight loss, or pain.

- Initial symptoms are nearly always followed up with a biopsy, where a piece of the tumor or potentially cancerous cells are analyzed by a pathologist, who verifies the diagnosis, identifies the type of cancer, and then assigns a stage to it. Those stages usually range from one to four, with four being the final, more advanced stage of cancer.

- Scientists tend to believe that an interaction of a number of different factors produce cancer. The factors involved might be a genetic risk or vulnerability. There might be viral factors, or it might be hormonal. It could involve environmental exposures to radiation or toxins, for example, or it might be behavioral and involve health-related behaviors like smoking, diet, sexual behavior, and exposure to ultraviolet radiation.

- One of the strongest risk factors is simply growing older. The longer you live, the more your cells divide, the more opportunities those cells have to make a mistake, and your immune system isn't able to capture it. The majority of cancers don't start until after people are 65 years or older.

Cancer Treatments
- In the realm of biomedical medicine, we have made some very impressive advancements in oncology (treating various cancers). Ultimately, when a patient is receiving treatment for cancer, it usually involves multiple categories used in sync with one another.

- The fist category is surgery. If a tumor is identified and is localized, then surgery may be curative. The goal of surgery is to remove all of the cancer. Surgery also might be palliative. If a tumor is pressing on your spinal cord and causing a great deal of pain or maybe even paralysis, you can't take all of the tumor out and cure the cancer, but you can ease some of the negative symptoms.

- The second category is radiation therapy, which involves essentially zapping the area with radiation. You kill healthy cells along with unhealthy cells. Of course, radiation has grown more advanced and

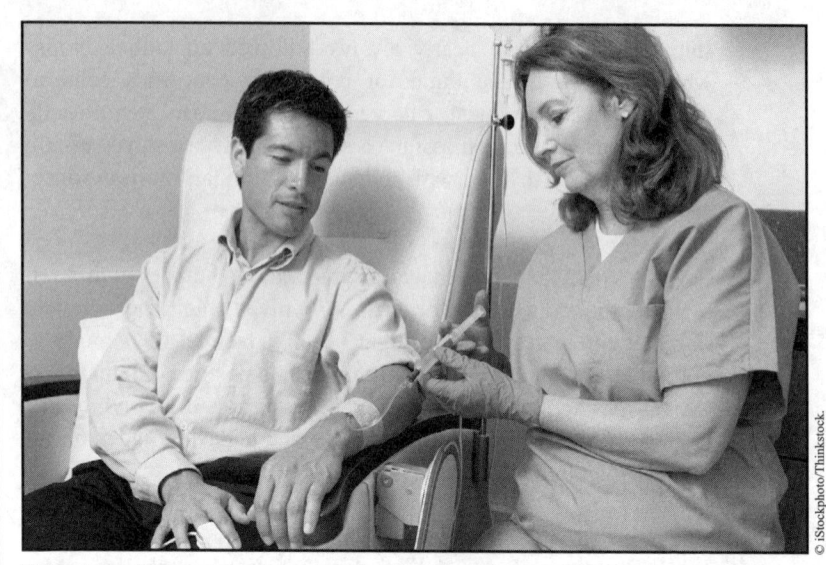

With chemotherapy, there is a vast array of drugs and delivery methods.

more localized, and there are different ways to deliver those bursts of specialized radiation.

- The third category is chemotherapy. This category is the largest vast array of drugs, and often, it's not just a single drug but multiple drugs or combinations of drugs. Different delivery methods might even be used. It can be systemically administered, or you could have actual pellets of medication inserted in particular parts of the body. Essentially, chemotherapy is a poison for cancer cells, but it also poisons the individual and has a great deal of side effects.

- The next category is hormone therapy. Some cancers grow faster as a consequence of stimulation from hormones. A hormone therapy would block the hormones that the cancer needs to continue to grow. Biologic therapies is an emerging field that looks at different biological agents, such as bacteria, to stimulate the body's own immune system in a way that will make it more effective in fighting cancer.

- The last category, which is still fairly new, is stem cell transplantation, which is currently used so that a patient can receive very high doses of chemotherapy or radiation. Those stem cells can then, for example, replenish bone marrow or blood products so that the individual is able to take higher and more intensive doses of treatment.

Stress and Social Support
- In terms of the biopsychosocial model, we would like to determine if any of the psychosocial factors—emotions, cognitions, personality, social relationships, identity, the power of place, and socioeconomic status—play a role in the etiology, or onset, of cancer and whether psychosocial treatments could affect cancer outcomes.

- We can consider stress to be both a potential cause of cancer and an almost definite consequence of cancer. Even if we decide that there's not a causal link, it doesn't mean that we shouldn't consider stress or stress management as part of a treatment program.

- Is stress related to cancer onset? The literature is fairly vast. Some studies look at stress and initial onset. Some studies look at stress and the progression of cancer. Others look at stress as a potential cause of the recurrence of cancer after treatment has ended.

- There are many different kinds of cancer that can be in nearly any different bodily system or organ, so the role that stress may play in lung cancer versus prostate cancer, for example, may vary.

- In addition, some cancers are more sensitive to hormonal fluctuations. Some cancers are more sensitive to contraction of a virus. Some of these might be more or less sensitive to stress.

- The research on stress and cancer, at least in humans, is so far contradictory and inconclusive. Stress seems to play some role, but a direct cause-effect relationship between stress and cancer onset has not been proven.

- Stronger evidence does link stress and cancer progression, so even if stress doesn't cause cancer, once you have it, stress may play an important role in causing that cancer to progress. It's unclear, though, how big of a role this might be.

- It's nearly impossible to look at stress alone without the presence of other factors that could be influencing progressions, such as genetic vulnerability, diet, smoking, or the environment. The biopsychosocial model gives us a rich, interdependent, complex look at diseases, but it's very difficult to tease individual causal elements apart.

- Even if we aren't able to ultimately prove that stress is a causal factor in the onset or progression of cancer, stress management in the treatment is undeniably beneficial in improving mood, outlook, relationships, and quality of life.

- Stress management, even if it turns out that it doesn't have that large of a role in terms of cancer biology, should be part of any comprehensive treatment package.

- Social support raises the same questions as stress: Is it linked to the onset or progression of cancer? Can it affect treatment or outcomes?

- In 2007, the Institute of Medicine released a report on psychosocial aspects of cancer care. They noted that all cancer treatment should assist the patient with pain, depression, anxiety, side effects of treatment, coping with stress, life adjustments, and spiritual counseling. They should also assist the family with distress, caregiving tasks, respite, finances, and spiritual counseling.

Suggested Reading

Institute of Medicine, *Cancer Care for the Whole Patient*.

Martz and Livneh, *Coping with Chronic Illness and Disability*.

Satterfield, *Minding the Body.*

Spiegel, Bloom, Kraemer, and Gottheil, "Effect of Psychosocial Treatment on Survival of Patients with Metastatic Breast Cancer."

Questions to Consider

1. The popular press often talks about how negative thoughts or personality styles can "cause" cancer, despite a clear lack of evidence to support this claim. Why do these claims persist? What negative impacts might these false claims have?

2. What advice would you have for a patient with advanced cancer who wants to try a controversial and possibly harmful treatment? Wouldn't you try everything possible? At what point should one transition from curative to palliative care?

Bugs, Drugs, and Buddha—Psychoneuroimmunology
Lecture 27

In this lecture, you will learn about immunology and disease. You will combine what you have learned about the immunology pathway with your knowledge of psychological and social factors to understand chronic diseases, such as HIV/AIDS and asthma. You will also use what you have learned about stress, coping, behavior, relationships, and the social environment. In addition, you will learn about interventions to improve or recalibrate the immune system, some of which seem to effectively improve immune functioning.

Chronic Diseases: HIV/AIDS

- There are three key elements of wound healing: We need to fight off infections, we need some level of inflammation to promote healing, and we need tissue reconstruction. Stress can make us susceptible to the common cold, and it can dramatically slow the wound-healing process. Stress management plays an important part in wound healing and recovery from surgery.

- Both human immunodeficiency virus (HIV) and asthma are chronic diseases that involve aberrations in the immune system. With HIV, we see a particularly vicious virus decimating the normal immune system and making the host vulnerable to all sorts of opportunistic infections. With asthma, we have an overly sensitive and overly vigorous immune response that causes sometimes severe and even fatal inflammation and closure of the airways.

- Acquired immunodeficiency syndrome (AIDS) is caused by a retrovirus, HIV, which attacks helper T cells and affects macrophages in the immune system.

- HIV is primarily contracted through the exchange of bodily fluids, especially semen and blood. It has a variable incubation rate—for reasons that we don't entirely understand—while it's doing its work of essentially wiping out T cells and macrophages and severely damaging the immune system.

- Eventually, HIV progresses to AIDS, which has been officially defined as having HIV and a helper T cell count of less than 200. According to the Centers for Disease Control, over 1 million people in the United States are HIV positive. Worldwide, that number is about 34 million, with the majority of cases in sub-Saharan Africa.

- In 1996, anti-retroviral medications were discovered, and the drug cocktail—which was eventually responsible for saving hundreds of thousands of lives and is now the mainstay of treatment for HIV suppression, although not yet eradication, around the world— was born.

- Many of our current efforts include both treatment and prevention. There is also a behavioral campaign to promote safe sex and prevent the transmission of HIV.

- In general, we know that the effects of chronic stress speed the progression of AIDS and predict more opportunistic infections. HIV attacks both T cells and macrophages, or frontline immunity, and chronic stress similarly hits both frontline and backline immunity in our interactive immune system.

- It seems that, conceptually, we have an explanation and some interesting, tantalizing studies. It seems logical, then, that stress reduction interventions might slow HIV and prolong survival—but that's not what we've found over decades of research.

- It seems that stress reduction definitely improves mental health and quality of life. Some studies show improvement in immune system parameters, but these statistically significant differences have not translated into clinical improvements or longer survival.

- For now, the bottom line—as described in the 2008 meta-analysis by Lori Scott-Sheldon looking at 46 different stress-reduction interventions—is that stress reduction works for anxiety, depression, distress, fatigue, and quality of life. It does not, however, alter helper T cell counts or hormonal measures in a meaningful way in order to extend survival.

Chronic Diseases: Asthma

- Like HIV/AIDS, asthma is also immunologically mediated and influenced by stress. Although asthma is not as prevalent as HIV/AIDS and doesn't have as high of a mortality rate, it is still important.

- Asthma is a chronic lung disease in which inflammation causes your airways to narrow. It's not technically an autoimmune disease, but it can be severe and disabling.

- There are a number of different subtypes of asthma. The main type is called allergic, or atopic, asthma, which makes up about 90 percent of asthma cases.

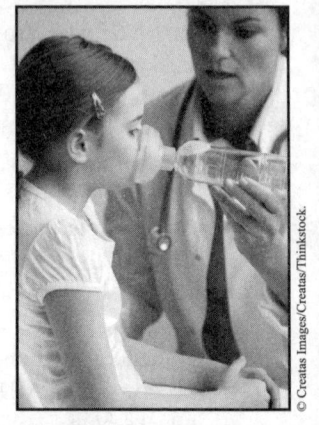

About 26 million people in the United States have asthma.

- Allergic asthma is triggered by an allergic reaction to antigens or allergens, such as pollen or pet dander. If you have allergic asthma, you probably have a personal and/or family history of allergies, such as allergic rhinitis or hay fever and/or eczema.

- There are two basic kinds of medication for treating asthma: Control drugs are used to prevent attacks from occurring, and quick relief, or rescue, drugs are used during attacks. The most common is a corticosteroid inhaler, which is similar to cortisol and causes the inflammation in the lungs to go down.

- If we view asthma through a biopsychosocial lens, we see a number of important factors. The social environmental might expose you to particular environmental triggers. The physical environment will also matter: Is it a dirty environment with a lot of allergens, such as pets or cigarette smoke? In terms of psychological variables, there are behaviors that might expose you to other allergens.

- Does stress serve as a trigger for an asthma attack? Studies looking at college students before an exam have found that stressed-out college students with asthma have a drop in their FEV1, which is the forced expiratory volume of air, or how much air they can breathe out in one second. It's a very common, simple, and cheap way to measure pulmonary function.

- However, it's important to remember that even though you have a blip in terms of intensity of stress before an exam, many college students are chronically stressed out, and of course, they often don't have very good health-related behaviors either. It seems like there is some relationship between stress and asthma in asthmatic college students.

- In epidemiologic studies, having anxiety—being exposed to domestic violence or having violence in your childhood (for example, childhood abuse)—is linked to having asthma as a child but also as an adult.

- Social stressors, especially chronic social stressors, induce corticosteroid insensitivity, which in part may be a result of impaired glucocorticoid receptor expression and/or function. That's important because when we're stressed, HPA turns on and secretes cortisol. In the short term, it causes a decrease in inflammation and should actually help your asthma.

- If a person has chronic social stress, cortisol loses the ability to cause that decrease in inflammation and no longer helps. In fact, it actually starts to hurt. We also know that interventions to reduce stress can improve lung function in asthma outcomes.

- Cortisol typically suppresses inflammation, but this isn't what we see with asthma. It gets more confusing if you think about our other stress-response system, sympathetic adrenal medullary system, which releases epinephrine and norepinephrine. One of the effects of epinephrine is bronchodilation. If you have cortisol, which suppresses inflammation, and you have epinephrine, which opens up your airways, why is it that stress makes asthma worse?

- This is called the asthma paradox. With chronic stress, we see glucocorticoid receptor insensitivity. Essentially, cortisol loses its abilities to suppress inflammation. When you take a corticosteroid inhaler, the amount of cortisol-like drug that you are taking is so large that it's able to overcome that amount of insensitivity.

- This insensitivity theory is something similar that's happening with your beta-adrenergic receptors that are typically stimulated by epinephrine. If you're in a chronically stressed-out state, your epinephrine stays high and those beta-adrenergic receptors become insensitive.

- On the other hand, research regarding an acute stressor and the onset of an asthma attack shows the existence of a fairly robust relationship. Acute stress, or short-term stress, can cause a person to have an asthma attack. This doesn't seem to match our model, but if you look a little more closely, you'll see that acute stress triggers an attack in people who are already chronically stressed.

- Most of these studies are done with children who are in underserved populations and high-stress environments. They're exposed to an acute stressor or an environmental trigger—some sort of allergen, for example—and that acute stress is enough to cause an asthma attack to occur, probably in people who are already chronically stressed to begin with.

Improving Immunity
- To improve our immunity, we want to look at stress management. We want to look at tailored cognitive behavioral therapy that can target fatigue, function, and maybe depression and can help us accept medical problems that we might have.

- Jim Pennebaker has researched expressive writing for patients with asthma and rheumatoid arthritis. By writing about a stressful event, by essentially purging that event out of them and putting it on paper, patients had improved outcomes with both asthma and rheumatoid arthritis.

- Mindfulness meditation is another way to manage stress. If an individual is practicing mindfulness meditation and they get a flu shot, they have a more robust immune antibody response to that flu shot.

- In general, the relationship between physical activity and the immune system is sort of U-shaped. If you do not have any physical activity, it is not so great for your immune system. If you have too much physical activity that involves putting a lot of wear and tear on your body, your immune system is actually suppressed. Of course, it depends on frequency, intensity, and physical conditioning.

Suggested Reading

Davidson, et al, "Alterations in Brain and Immune Function Produced by Mindfulness Meditation."

Martz and Livneh, *Coping with Chronic Illness and Disability*.

Sapolsky, *Why Zebras Don't Get Ulcers*.

Satterfield, *Minding the Body*.

Questions to Consider

1. Given that stress serves an important evolutionary function—namely, to marshal resources to either fight or flee—why does stress suppress the immune system? Wouldn't that be disadvantageous?

2. The prevalence of food allergies has been rising dramatically over the past decade. Are there mind-body or other factors that might account for this?

Fire in the Belly—The GI System
Lecture 28

We know from personal experience that the mind and gut are somehow related, but now with our understanding of the biopsychosocial model—and especially our stress-response systems—we can start deepening what we know about how and why stress influences our gastrointestinal (GI) system in both good and bad ways. This lecture will review the digestive system, including common symptoms of diseases and their causes. You will also learn about two different stress-related GI disorders, ulcers and irritable bowel syndrome, to further explore this mind-gut connection.

The Anatomy and Physiology of the GI System

- Simply put, digestion is the use of both chemical and mechanical means to break food into small, usable molecules. Given the complexity of what we eat, we need a variety of enzymes and digestive juices to effectively extract all of the nutrients from our food as it passes on its way through our alimentary canal—from the mouth all the way to the anus.

- Food is moved through this highly efficient and impressive system primarily through peristalsis, or waves of muscle contractions that push the food continuously forward.

- The mouth has both mechanical and chemical digestive elements. Chewing is the mechanical breakdown of food. Saliva, with its digestive enzymes, is our first chemical attempt to start breaking down starches and other foods to ease digestion a little bit later. Our first digestive glands are our salivary glands.

- Once the voluntary action of swallowing has been initiated, our esophagus, which is essentially just a tube, allows food to travel from our mouth down to our stomach, where both mechanical and chemical digestion occur.

- Right before the food gets to the stomach, we have an esophageal sphincter. It's usually closed. When food touches the top of it, it will open so that food can drop down into the stomach.

- The stomach essentially has three mechanical tasks: to store food and liquid, to mix the food with various digestive juices, and to slowly empty its contents into the small intestines. The stomach slowly pushes food down to the next stop in the alimentary canal, the small intestines.

- The length of time that food spends in the stomach is affected by a number of different variables, including the type of food that you consume. Carbohydrates, and especially simple carbohydrates, are digested the quickest and spend the least amount of time in the stomach. Proteins stay in the stomach longer, and fats stay in the stomach the longest.

- Chemical digestion occurs from both hydrochloric acid, or stomach acid, and a soup of different enzymes that are within the stomach. The stomach keeps from digesting itself with the help of a protective mucosal lining. This lining constantly needs to be replenished, and a number of factors can weaken this lining so that the stomach acid actually begins to burn the inside of the stomach.

- The most common symptom is heartburn. If it occurs chronically it's called gastroesophageal reflux disorder. Nearly everyone experiences this at some point, and 20 percent of the population experiences it weekly—hence the incredible market for medications like Prilosec or over-the-counter medications like Zantac or Tums.

- After exiting the stomach, your food, or whatever is left of it, enters the small intestines—or, specifically, the duodenum, where enzymes from the pancreas, liver, and intestines further break down food molecules. Which enzymes are used depends on what kind of food you ate and how much you consumed.

- At this point in the process, your body is essentially trying to break down the food into its simplest molecular constituents so that it can use whatever nutrients you might need. The rest is just going to past through.

- Our liver primarily produces bile, which is stored in our gallbladder, and it is released to aid in the digestion of fats. This molecular soup is then slowly passed through the small intestines, and as this happens, there are millions of tiny fingerlike projections called villi, which have finger-like projections on them called microvilli that scoop through the molecular soup and pull through the nutrients that our body needs.

- Anything that's left over at the end of this complex process—such as fiber, for example—is considered waste. It goes on to the colon or the large intestines, where water and salt are reabsorbed. Whatever is left over after that reabsorption process is considered waste, which expelled whenever you have a bowel movement.

Stress and Digestion

- Gastrin causes the stomach to produce acid and is necessary to promote the growth of the lining of the stomach and the small intestines.

- Secretin stimulates enzyme production by the pancreas, bile from the liver, and causes the stomach to make an enzyme called pepsin.

- Cholecystokinin turns on the pancreas to produce enzymes and causes the gallbladder to release bile, or empty.

- Ghrelin is a hormone that's produced by the stomach and the upper intestines, and it stimulates hunger. *H. pylori* pushes down the levels of ghrelin.

- Leptin is produced by fat tissue, or white adipose tissue. It's released into the bloodstream and causes us to feel full.

- Each of these characters might prove important in helping us understand how psychological and social factors influence our GI health, such as how stress is related to obesity, how depression is linked to diabetes, or how brain chemistry contributes to eating disorders.

- Stress shuts down blood flow, decreases muscle contractions, and decreases digestive secretions. This is important for GI motility.

- In addition, recall that the mucosal lining of the stomach that prevents ulcers from forming needs to be replenished constantly. In order for it to be replenished, it has to have a robust blood supply. If that's being cut off or decreased because of stress, the mucosal lining is not being replenished as often as it needs to be.

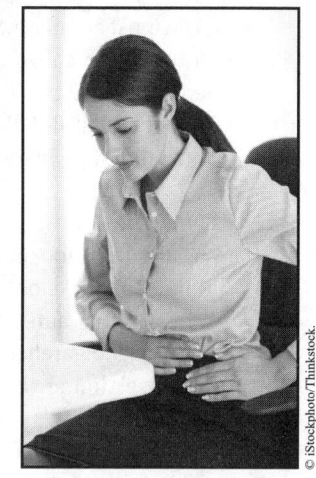

Stress has a negative effect on the digestive process.

- Stress can also cause inflammation of the gastrointestinal system, making you more susceptible to infections. Acute stress slows gastric emptying, but it speeds up colonic transit, resulting in diarrhea.

- Also, stress can play a role in dyspeptic, or heartburn, symptoms and alterations in stool frequency and consistency, which could mean constipation or diarrhea.

Ulcers and IBS

- A peptic ulcer is a defect in the lining of the stomach or in the first part of the small intestines, the area called the duodenum. A peptic ulcer in the stomach is called a gastric ulcer, and one in the duodenum is called a duodenal ulcer.

- The most common cause of ulcers—in 70 to 90 percent of cases—is a bacterium called *Helicobacter pylori*, or *H. pylori*. Many people are colonized by *H. pylori* and don't go on to develop an ulcer. It is possible that the ulcer forms as a result of *H. pylori* plus stress or the ratio of *H. pylori* to other flora or fauna that live in the gut.

- Other factors that might contribute are behavioral factors, such as drinking too much alcohol, which also weakens the mucosal lining of the stomach. In addition, the regular use of aspirin or nonsteroidal anti-inflammatory drugs, such as ibuprofen or Advil; smoking cigarettes, and chewing tobacco have an effect on the mucosal lining. Stress also plays a contributing role by altering blood flow.

- The primary treatment for ulcers is medication. There are two kinds of medications that will eradicate *H. pylori*. However, we're starting to wonder if complete eradication is actually a good thing.

- The first kind of medication increases the levels of ghrelin. None of the studies in this area have shown that *H. pylori* eradication is linked to subsequent weight gain and obesity, but maybe we just don't know yet.

- The other kind of medication is proton-pump inhibitors that lower the amount of stomach acid. The problem with these drugs is that once you're on them, it's hard to come off.

- Essentially, your stomach gets used to having an external crutch that's going to decrease the stomach acid, and it stops being so good at protecting itself. Once you come off of a proton-pump inhibitor, your stomach is very sensitive, and you actually get worse symptoms or rebound symptoms of dyspepsia or heartburn.

- Other treatments for ulcers include dietary or behavioral changes. Cutting out alcohol, smoking, and nonsteroidal anti-inflammatory drugs is important. In addition, stress management has been shown to be helpful.

- Irritable bowel syndrome (IBS) is a common GI issue that mostly occurs in the large intestine or the colon. IBS involves cramping, pain, bloating, diarrhea, and constipation. It doesn't cause permanent damage to the colon, although it can cause a lot of functional impairment.

- About 20 percent of people have had irritable bowel symptoms. It's more common in women than in men, and the onset tends to be before the age of 35. We don't know exactly what causes it, but we know that it's related to immune changes and how they affect the colon and GI motility.

- There is a theory about serotonin receptors and the level of serotonin. Most of us think of serotonin as related to depression, meaning that it occurs primarily in the brain. Actually, 95 percent of our serotonin is in our gut, and only 5 percent is in the brain.

- Patients with irritable bowel syndrome either have abnormal amounts of serotonin or receptors that aren't working properly. They will either increase GI motility, meaning that things move through the colon too quickly and you get diarrhea, or they move too slowly and you get constipation.

- Fortunately, the prognosis for IBS is quite good. IBS is rarely severe, and it can be managed with diet and sometimes with medications.

- In terms of GI motor activity, stress shuts down muscle contractions. If this occurs before the colon, it means that things aren't going to move forward, delaying gastric emptying. But if this occurs after the colon, it means that things are going to move out more quickly, meaning that you're more likely to get diarrhea.

- In addition to dietary changes and some limited support from medication, treatment for depression, anxiety, and stress reduction can all improve IBS symptoms.

- At this point, few would say that stress causes IBS or that stress management cures it, but it can certainly play an important role, as we've seen with a number of other diseases as well.

Suggested Reading

Martz and Livneh, *Coping with Chronic Illness and Disability*.

Satterfield, *Minding the Body*.

Spector, "Germs Are Us."

Questions to Consider

1. George Engel's experience with baby Monica taught us that stress slows or stops the digestive process. If that's true, why do we think stress contributes to ulcers? Wouldn't stress lower stomach acid and other secretions?

2. How might medicine harness the "microbiome" to manage obesity or gastrointestinal conditions like irritable bowel syndrome or ulcerative colitis? What would a treatment look like?

Obesity—America's New Epidemic
Lecture 29

In this lecture, you will explore the phenomenon of overnutrition—better known as being overweight or obese. You will learn about the health ramifications and the epidemiology of obesity. You will also learn about the effects of stress, social factors, and behavioral factors on weight gain. Obesity is a global epidemic. In this lecture, you will discover some biopsychosocial interventions that might help people lose weight and get this epidemic under control.

Weight Issues

- Body mass index (BMI) is a person's weight in kilograms divided by his or her height in meters squared. If your BMI is between 25 and 30, you're considered overweight. If it's above 30, you are considered obese. If it's above 40, you are considered morbidly obese.

- Many have complained that BMI is perhaps a little too insensitive. It casts a rather wide net and captures a number of individuals that might not actually have a weight problem. For example, if you are a weightlifter and you have a lot of muscle mass, your BMI might actually place you in the overweight range.

- The alternative to using BMI is the waist-to-hip ratio, or the gut-to-butt ratio, which should be less than 0.95 for men and less than 0.80 for women.

- There is good evidence that links obesity to a number of different health problems. For example, being obese quadruples your risk of having diabetes, increases your risk for having high blood pressure by a factor of 5.6 times, more than doubles your risk for having high cholesterol, and increases the risk for cardiovascular disease and stroke.

- Poor diet and exercise has been linked to 25 percent of cancers. It's also linked to osteoarthritis, heartburn, and gastroesophageal reflux disorder. Recent evidence even shows us that obesity is linked to depression and earlier onset of Alzheimer's disease.

Biological Factors
- A potential biological explanation for obesity is genetics. The genetics explanation has a lot of appeal for many people because it matches what we've observed in the real world. Obesity tends to run in families. It might also give us a much-needed break from all of the blaming that often accompanies discussions of weight.

- From twin studies, adoption studies, and animal studies, the genetically determined contribution to obesity is believed to lie somewhere between 25 and 40 percent, which leaves 60 plus percent from something else.

- The Institute of Medicine and the World Health Organization conclude that although genetics is important, the environment is the largest single influence on body weight.

- Energy balance is the key to regulation of body weight. This involves calories taken in versus calories burned off. It isn't really that simple because our rate of energy expenditure, or our metabolism, may changes over time.

- Metabolic rate slows with age. Beginning in our mid-20s, we lose about one-third of a percent of muscle mass by weight each year for the rest of our lives—unless, of course, we're doing things to build muscle.

- With that five percent decline per decade in basal metabolic rate, it reduces the number of calories that we need to maintain our weight. Unfortunately, as we get older, we don't typically lower our caloric intake, leading to our weight eventually creeping up over time.

- Some people have argued that our aging population's slowing metabolic rate is the reason that we're seeing part of the increase in the rates of obesity and overweight people. It's not enough to account for the big changes that we've seen over the past few decades, but it might be part of the explanation.

- Fat is the largest endocrine organ that we have in our body. It is metabolically active—not just a storage device. Fat secretes chemicals, including leptin, which is responsible for giving us a sense of satiety. Unfortunately, if you have a lot of fat cells secreting a lot of leptin, you develop leptin insensitivity.

Social and Environmental Influences

- In terms of social and environmental influences, there are familial and cultural linkages to food and eating behaviors. Food is often a way to express love or nurturance. It is a way for us to demonstrate respect for tradition or for holidays.

- Of course, those familial and cultural influences occur in a broader environment that further influence our choices. That broader environment includes things like socioeconomic status and the food environment of your neighborhood.

- More broadly, many people have been looking at what they have called the toxic food environment. We're often influenced to make bad choices. Maybe those choices about food are because of our toxic food environment.

- Depressingly, a quarter of the vegetable consumption in the United States is french fries. In addition, portion sizes have changed increased over the past 20 or 30 years.

- Of course, other influences have to do with marketing—especially marketing that is targeted at children, a particularly vulnerable population. The average time a child spends watching TV amounts to about 10,000 TV ads throughout their childhood, and 95 percent of those ads are for sugary cereals, soda, candy, and fast food. In addition, we're serving them fast food at school, and we don't give them a chance to exercise.

Stress and Obesity

- Stress affects the food choices that we make, but it also affects whether we choose to be physically active. Most of us do not reach for a salad when we're stressed. In fact, 65 percent of us reach for candy or chocolate, and 56 percent of us reach for more ice cream when we're stressed.

- Only 14 percent of people eat fruit when they're stressed, and 8 percent eat vegetables. Of course, it's partly culture, but it might also be brain chemistry, which links us back to biology.

- To date, nearly 40 studies have looked at the biological addictive potential of food. Some people do genuinely develop addiction to food (think of binge eating disorders). For most of us, though, our brain tricks us into eating more than intended and into making worse food choices than planned.

- Our mesolimbic reward pathways are activated by junk foods or foods that we enjoy. Consequently, we're compelled to make bad choices. We can still choose otherwise, but the deck is stacked against us.

- Given that we're in essence fighting against our history and against our mesolimbic dopamine pathways, we could think of public health interventions that might reengineer food availability. We might consciously think about developing new habits in the ways that we respond to stress or try to limit our exposures to bad food.

- We might try stress reduction as an alternative to managing our moods, other than reaching for junk foods. We need to sleep more when we are stressed instead of sleeping less, which is what most people do. We need to develop the habit of exercising when we're stressed; it's a remarkably potent stress tool, but most of us exercise less when we're stressed instead of more.

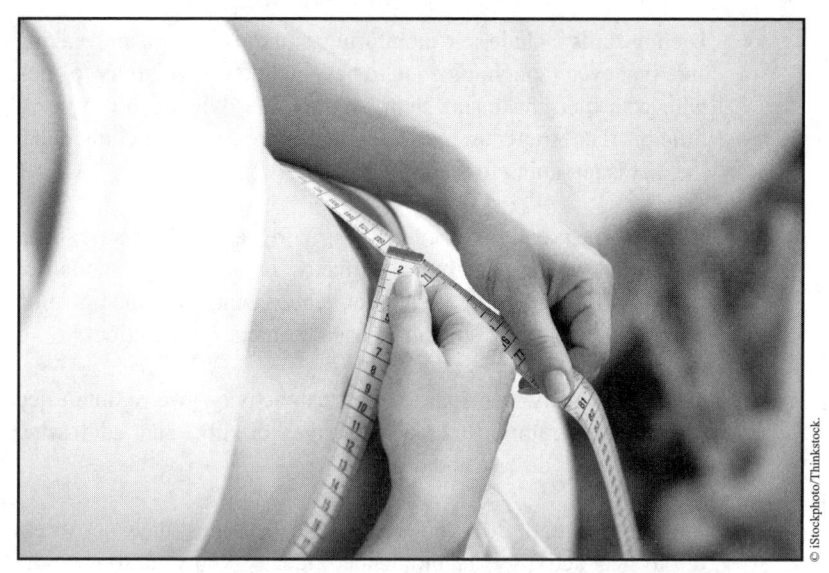

One way to manage your weight is to not buy junk foods in the first place.

Weight Management

- Weight management is a multibillion-dollar industry. When we talk about diets, we're usually talking about reduction in calories and weight management. We might also be talking about simply improving nutrition even if the caloric count stays the same.

- Because our metabolic rate changes, we probably also want to think about an increase in physical activity. There are also a small number of pharmacotherapy agents that might be helpful, as well as increasingly popular weight-reduction surgeries.

- The first thing we can do to help with weight management is set realistic initial goals. We want to be as fit as possible at our current weight and prevent further weight gain. If we're successful at the first two, then maybe we can think about weight loss.

- Dieting skills include self-monitoring, stimulus control, and making sure that even though it's good to have willpower and to try to stick with your diet, make sure that there are days when you can flex a little bit. The stricter an individual is, the greater the likelihood that the diet is not going to work.

- Medical interventions include gastric bypass and gastric band surgeries. These are enormously effective in losing large amounts of weight, but they do require a great deal of behavioral modification after the surgery. Liposuction is just a cosmetic intervention.

- There are many benefits of physical activity. We're interested in cardiorespiratory fitness, reducing mortality, and addressing cardiovascular disease and other diseases.

- For the most part, 30 to 60 minutes per day, most days per week, of physical activity is recommended. Ideally, you want to try to be at 60 to 90 percent of your maximum heart rate for at least half an hour or so. Your maximum heart rate is about 220 minus your age.

Suggested Reading

Brownell, Kersh, Ludwig, Post, Puhl, Schwartz, and Willett, "Personal Responsibility and Obesity."

Gardner, Kiazand, Alhassan, et al, "Comparison of the Atkins, Zone, Ornish, and LEARN Diets for Change in Weight and Related Risk Factors among Overweight Premenopausal Women."

Kessler, *The End of Overeating*.

Martz and Livneh, *Coping with Chronic Illness and Disability*.

Satterfield, *Minding the Body*.

Questions to Consider

1. What are the advantages and disadvantages of classifying obesity as a disease or as an addiction? What are the social and psychological ramifications?

2. What interventions hold the greatest promise for getting the obesity epidemic under control? How much will it cost? How much should we pay?

The Strain in Pain Lies Mainly in the Brain
Lecture 30

In this lecture, you will learn about the basics of acute pain and chronic pain and how mind-body factors can play a critical role in both the cause and treatment of chronic pain conditions. You will learn how pain is measured. You will also learn about the pathophysiology of pain and the role of the central nervous system, for example, in the role of phantom limb pain. In addition, you will examine mind-body factors in chronic pain, and you will learn about biopsychosocial treatments for pain, including different kinds of psychotherapy, acupuncture, mindfulness-based stress reduction, and biofeedback.

Acute versus Chronic Pain

- The International Association for the Study of Pain defines pain as an unpleasant sensory and emotional experience associated with actual or potential tissue damage.

- In general, acute pain is thought to be an important and adaptive signal. It tells us of imminent or ongoing tissue damage. It also increases the likelihood of single-trial learning—which is the proverbial hot stove that you learn right away not to touch.

- The process of being able to feel pain is called nociception. There are four basic steps. The first step is transduction, which is where nociceptors, or pain receptors, transduce noxious stimuli into nociceptive impulses.

- The second step is transmission, where electrical impulses are sent via afferent nerves to the spinal cord, then along sensory tracts to the brain.

- The third step is modulation, which is the process of either dampening or amplifying a pain signal related to the neural signal. This is hugely important when we think about mind-body factors in

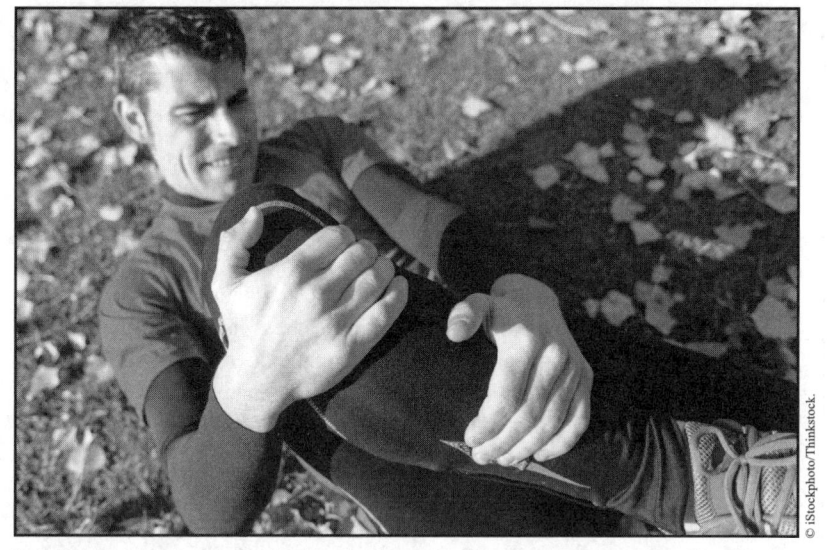

Pain is not just about physical sensation; it's also about the mind and body.

pain because we know that people modulate, often unconsciously, the pain that they are experiencing. We know that it can happen in both the spinal cord as well as in the brain.

- The fourth step is pain perception, which is the subjective experience of pain that results from transduction, transmission, and modulation plus the psychological and social factors that are at play. This is our brain at work, often altering what it is that we are perceiving.

- Chronic pain has usually been defined arbitrarily as pain that persists for three to six months or longer—or even beyond the period of expected healing. Ongoing or progressive tissue damage may be present in some types of chronic pain, including progressive neuropathic pain and rheumatologic conditions.

- In other cases, though, chronic pain may be present even when tissue damage is stable or has been undetected. Unlike acute pain, chronic pain is now thought to be a disease of the central nervous system that involves some sort of maladaptive reprogramming of the brain and/or the spinal cord.

- The brain can generate terrible pain in a wound that has long been healed. It can even generate chronic pain in a limb that no longer exists.

- Acute pain, such as acute stress, has a function, and it helps us survive. Chronic pain, such as chronic stress, is an entirely different disorder. Chronic pain can have potentially devastating consequences on mood, cause depression and anger, damage social relationships, wreck finances, and have a large impact on self-image.

- Unfortunately, there's really no good objective measure of pain. There's no lab test, scan, or image that can help a medical professional, or even a patient or individual, know exactly objectively how much pain they are experiencing.

- In a medical setting, doctors will often ask the following: On a scale of 1 to 10—with 1 being no pain and 10 being the worst pain imaginable—how intense has your pain been? For children or people who don't understand the numeric scale, doctors use simple happy and sad faces, asking them to pick which face represents their level of pain.

- You might also be asked questions about functional impairment, which involves what your pain prevents you from doing. This could be impairment in activities of daily living, or it might be functional impairment in the context of social or occupational functioning.

Modulation and Perception

- Modulation is real. When soldiers are injured in the field, they often experience no pain. In addition, athletes who are in a race often don't realize that they might have injured themselves.

- Phantom limb pain in upper-limb amputations happens over 80 percent of the time. There are a number of different treatments that have been tried to treat a limb that isn't there, including applying electrodes to the stump of the amputated limb and injecting analgesics into the stump of the amputated limb or into the spinal cord and actually doing nerve blocks.

- In response to the growing awareness of mind-body phenomenon in the realm of pain, the gate control theory of pain was described in the early 1960s by Ron Melzack and Patrick Wall. In this theory, pain signals encounter what they call nerve gates in the spinal cord that open or close, depending on a number of factors, possibly including instructions that might be coming down from the brain to the spinal cord.

- These gates would open or close to increase, modulate, or decrease the sensation of pain. When these gates are open, pain messages get through faster, and the pain can be quite intense. When the gates are closed, pain messages are prevented from reaching the brain and may not even be experienced or perceived.

- There are a number of observational studies on the variability of pain experience. Pain transmission seems to have a limited bandwidth.

- Positive or negative emotions might play a role. If an individual is placed in a positive mood, usually through watching videos or recalling favorite memories, he or she is able to tolerate pain for a longer period of time. In addition, if an individual is in a positive mood, he or she is able to tolerate a much stronger or intense sensation of pain than if in a negative mood. Perhaps this is due to the gate control theory.

Pain Management

- Pharmacotherapy involves drugs that for the most part are in the opioid family, such as morphine or hydrocodone, but there are a number of other medications that can be helpful for pain in different families. Opioids work because they are similar to our bodies' own pain relievers—the endogenous opiates.

- When it comes to treating pain, one size does not fit all. Usually, you want a toolbox of different interventions to manage your pain. Together with your health-care team, you want to find what the best pain management package is for you.

- One of the early core skills of patient self-management is self-monitoring, where you're essentially gathering data on yourself. You might want to create a pain diary, where you collect data about your pain experience. In addition to noting details about your pain, you want to record any interventions that you've tried and assess whether they've helped or worked.

- A pain management package would include things like practical, structural, or mechanical interventions. This would include things like physical therapy and environmental changes. It also might include things like braces or wraps or using ice, heat, or even massage. These are all in the practical or mechanical category.

- In the psychological category, we want to use some cognitive strategies, including cognitive behavioral therapy, focusing on expectations and attitudes.

- We want patients to challenge maladaptive habits. We want them to challenge those catastrophizing thoughts, including thinking about things in all-or-none terms and maximizing or minimizing. We want them to think about either distraction on one hand or mindfulness on the other.

- There are also behavioral strategies for pain management, including massage and physical therapy. This might also include physical exercise. When people are in pain, it often hurts to exercise, but that's exactly what a physical therapist wants to do—usually through graded physical activity, which is one of the best interventions.

- In the world of complementary and alternative medicine, the first intervention is acupuncture, whose primary goal is to assess and rebalance the life force of the individual. This life force is known as Chi, which is located and flows throughout meridians of the body.

- In acupuncture, it is believed that the stimulation of certain points of the meridians with small inserted needles helps to rebalance the body. Perhaps nociceptors are being stimulated, and maybe the body is being told to release endogenous opiates.

- The evidence is considered strong for the efficacy of acupuncture in postoperative pain and in chemotherapy nausea and vomiting. Meta-analyses have found evidence that acupuncture is effective for pain relief for lower back pain and is much better than sham acupuncture or no additional treatment.

- Mindfulness-based stress reduction (MBSR), developed by Jon Kabat-Zinn, is a combination of mindfulness meditation and yoga. MBSR is a group program that usually lasts 8 to 10 weeks and involves one two-and-a-half-hour session per week. It's not spiritually based, but mindfulness does seem to have fairly deep Buddhist roots.

- MBSR is helpful for chronic pain—even in low-income, underserved populations, where typically many interventions don't work quite as well. It also works for decreasing lower back pain, coping with pain in general, decreasing stress, improving mood, and even increasing immune function.

- Biofeedback is usually some sort of often visual feedback from a biological monitoring device or computer that gives you information about a physiological process. It might tell you how tense your neck muscles are or give you information on skin temperature or blood pressure. Your job is simply to look at the needle or graph and make it move simply by thinking about it.

- The research supports that biofeedback actually works. In fact, there's something about the visual stimulus that gives people a sense of control and self-efficacy—belief that they can do something about it. The strongest evidence is in biofeedback for headaches and migraines.

Suggested Reading

Caudill-Slosberg, *Managing Pain Before It Manages You*.

Kabat-Zinn, *Full Catastrophe Living*.

Martz and Livneh, *Coping with Chronic Illness and Disability*.

Satterfield, *Minding the Body*.

Questions to Consider

1. Given the power of the placebo response in affecting pain, how can we harness it to provide a drug-free method of reducing pain? Doesn't this imply that pain is all in our heads and should be within our control?

2. Do mind-body pain interventions like hypnosis, biofeedback, meditation, or yoga all work through similar pathways? Would doing more than one at a time yield greater benefits than doing one alone?

Catching Your Zs—Sleep and Health
Lecture 31

Despite centuries of interest in the topic, there's actually quite a lot we don't know about sleep. In fact, we don't know for certain why we sleep or what the functions of sleep are, but we do know that sleep is important. In this lecture, you will learn what normal sleep is, in terms of both quantity and quality. You will also learn about the different stages of sleep, or sleep architecture. In addition, you will learn about the causes and possible treatments for insomnia.

The Facts about Sleep

- On average, people need about seven to eight hours of sleep per night, but there is some variability between individuals. Sleep is organized into five sleep stages that are systematically spread across the time that we are sleeping: stages 1, 2, 3, and 4 (non-REM sleep) and rapid eye movement (REM sleep).

- Each stage has a characteristic pattern on an electroencephalogram (EEG), which measures brain activity. In sleep studies, they may also use an electrooculogram (EOG), which measures eye movements and an electromyogram (EMG0), which measures muscle tension or muscle movements.

- Together, the EEG, EOG, and EMG are called a polysomnogram, and the practice of conducting these tests is called polysomnography. A polysomnogram will often generate a hypnogram, which is simply a graph of the quality of your night's sleep.

- A full cycle of all five stages is typically about 90 to 100 minutes. After you finish a full cycle, you start over. Depending on how long you sleep over the course of the night, you will have anywhere between four to six full cycles of all five stages of sleep.

- In general, in young and healthy adults, non-REM sleep—stages 1 through 4—accounts for about 75 to 90 percent of sleep time. We spend about 3 to 5 percent of our sleep time in stage 1, about 50 to 60 percent in stage 2, and about 10 to 20 percent in stages 3 and 4. Our REM sleep, when we believe we're dreaming, accounts for only about 10 to 25 percent of sleep time.

What Makes Us Sleep?

- There are two biological systems that make us sleep. The first is circadian rhythms, which is essentially our internal clock that gives us a sense of a day. Diurnal rhythms tell you when it's daytime and when it's nighttime, and they affect the flow of energy throughout the day.

- The second is the sleep homeostatic drive, which is some sort of innate pressure that forces us to sleep. If you have a bad night's sleep or if you stay up all night, the following day, even though your circadian rhythms tell you that it's daytime, your sleep homeostatic drive will be pushing you to follow sleep whenever it is possible.

- There are psychological factors that may also predispose us to sleep or not. We develop routines; we have scripts. There are things that we do right before bedtime that psychologically get us in the mindset that we are winding down.

- Mental fatigue, parasympathetic activation, and relaxation move us closer to sleep states. There are also a number of different social, cultural, and environmental factors. This has to do with your family responsibilities and your sleep environment. Is it quiet, or is it noisy?

Sleep Deprivation

- Animal studies have shown that sleep is necessary for survival. The normal life span of a rat is about two to three years. However, rats that were deprived of sleep live for only about three weeks. They also develop abnormally low body temperatures and sores on their tails and paws.

- Just getting a little bit less sleep is enough to affect your immune system so that it can increase your susceptibility to catching a cold or contracting a rhinovirus.

- In humans, it has been demonstrated that the metabolic activity of the brain decreases significantly after 24 hours of sustained wakefulness. Sleep deprivation results in a decrease in body temperature, immune system function as measured by the white blood cell count, and the release of growth hormones.

- Sleep deprivation can also cause changes in heart rate variability. It leads to impairment of memory, impaired physical performance, and reduced ability to carry out mathematical calculations. If sleep deprivation continues, hallucinations and mood swings may develop.

- Insomnia is a special kind of sleep deprivation. It is something that most of us have experienced acutely and some percentage of us experience chronically. Insomnia is defined as a difficulty with the initiation, maintenance, duration, or quality of sleep that results in the impairment of daytime functioning, despite adequate opportunity and circumstances for sleep.

- About 10 percent of the U.S. population has chronic insomnia, which is defined as insomnia lasting more than one month. Higher rates of insomnia occur in people with chronic pain, psychiatric disorders, and alcohol or drug addictions. The prevalence of insomnia generally rises with increased age.

- Causes of insomnia might include psychiatric disorders such as depression or anxiety and medical disorders such as chronic pain. They might include drugs—specifically, caffeine and alcohol.

- Other potential causes include psychophysiologic insomnia, which comes from somatized tension or worry or anxiety, which involves ruminating things in your head. Another cause could be circadian rhythm mismatch, of which jetlag and shift work are common examples.

- Another cause could be sleep state misperception. Sometimes patients will say that they haven't slept at all, but when they have a polysomnograph study done, it is discovered that they actually are sleeping, but they're dreaming that they're awake.

Sleep Management
- Sleep hygiene is a constellation of different behaviors that increase the likelihood that you'll be able to go to sleep. This includes keeping a regular bedtime and wake time (which means the same time on weekends as well as weekdays); keeping the bedroom quiet, comfortable, and dark; doing a relaxation technique for 10 to 20 minutes before you go to bed; getting regular exercise but not exercising right before bed; and not napping during the day.

- Do not lie in bed feeling worried, anxious, or frustrated. If you lie in bed for more than 30 minutes without falling asleep, get out of bed and do something that's relaxing. As soon as you feel sleepy, go back to bed. The idea is that you don't want to associate your bed with ruminating and feeling worried; instead, you want to associate your bed with feeling relaxed and comfortable and falling asleep.

- Limit the use of alcohol, caffeine, and even nicotine and other stimulants that can affect an individual's ability to go to sleep.

- Turn off the TV, cell phone, and computer. Interesting new research shows that by looking at one of those screens, it actually stimulates the sympathetic nervous system enough to make it more difficult for you to fall asleep.

- You could also use stimulus control therapy, which would involve going to bed early only when you are sleepy and getting up if you are ruminating.

- In addition, you could use sleep restriction therapy, where rather than tossing and turning for eight hours, if you usually get four hours of sleep per night, try to sleep for 4.5 hours. When you are

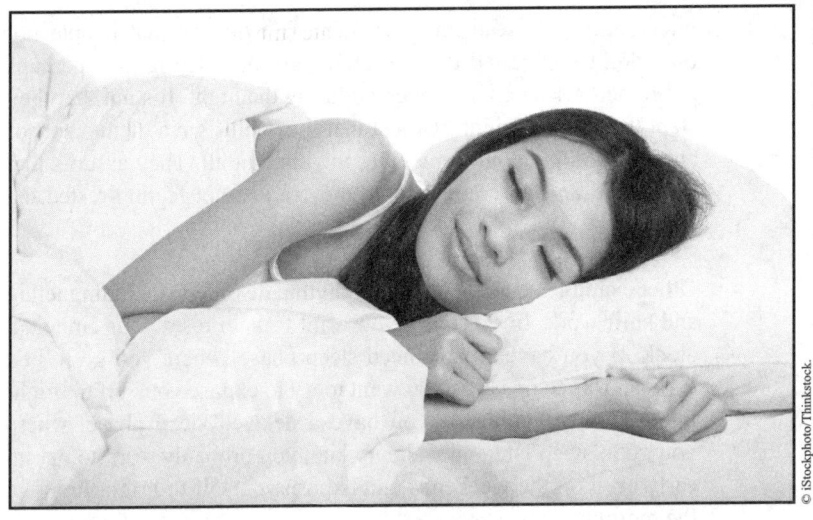

Many aspects of sleep are still unknown to science.

able to sleep for 4.5 hours, change it to five. Then, extend it to 5.5, and then six, and so on.

- You could try things like relaxation therapies, progressive muscle relaxations, and cognitive therapy. These work about 60 percent of the time, but that leaves about 40 percent of people who need something else.

- Most people turn to pharmacotherapy. There are a number of different medications that people can use. They're often called sedatives, hypnotics, or tranquilizers. They're in the category of benzodiazepines, such as Valium. There are newer benzodiazepine-like drugs, or agonists, such as Ambien, Sonata, and Lunesta. There are over-the-counter medications, such as diphenhydramine, which is Benadryl or the main ingredient in Tylenol PM. In addition, melatonin is an herbal approach.

- Unfortunately, even though people in general like sleep aids, there is no evidence that they work better than any cognitive behavioral interventions. Instead, there's emerging evidence that people not only don't feel rested the day afterward, but they're also perhaps not remembering what happened during the night. It's not that they slept through the night; it's just that those pills gave them a sort of amnesia so they don't remember the night at all. They assume that they slept, and for some reason, they're just not feeling rested the next day.

- Other examples include circadian rhythm disorders, including jetlag and shift work. In this case, you want to help reset your circadian clock. If you have an advanced sleep phase, where you go to bed early and wake up early, you want to try to expose yourself to bright lights in the evening. If you have a delayed sleep phase, where you go to sleep late and wake up late, you probably want to get up early even on the weekends and expose yourself to bright lights in the morning.

Suggested Reading

Jacobs, *Say Goodnight to Insomnia*.

Morin, Colecchi, Stone, Sood, and Brink, "Behavioral and Pharmacological Therapies for Late-Life Insomnia.

Satterfield, *Minding the Body*.

Questions to Consider

1. Sleep serves an essential restorative function necessary for health. But what functions do dreams serve? Are they symbolically meaningful or simply a "flush" of all the debris of the day? How can we answer that question?

2. Many studies have looked at the health consequences of not getting enough sleep, but what about getting too much sleep? How might too much sleep impact your health, and why?

Chasing Zebras—Somatoform Disorders
Lecture 32

In this lecture on somatization, you will learn about the full range of mind-body manifestations—from the very common complaint of fatigue to stress-related headaches to the family of psychiatric disorders called somatoform disorders. The goal is not to dismiss or disprove these conditions but, rather, to help us understand and to treat them more effectively. In this lecture, you will learn about some of the common somatic symptoms that occur in a primary care clinic. You will also contrast these common symptoms with the less common family of psychiatric disorders known as somatoform disorders.

Somatoform Disorders

- Fatigue is one of the most common symptoms that we see in primary care, followed by headaches, lower back pain, dizziness, insomnia, and widespread musculoskeletal pain. In more cases than not, there's no organic cause or diagnosis. Most are not linked to any particular disease. Most are put in the category of medically unexplained symptoms.

- In contrast, there is a range of psychiatric disorders called somatoform disorders that are much more intense versions of what the typical patient brings in.

- The term "somatization" refers to the experience and reporting of physical symptoms that cause distress but lack a corresponding level of tissue damage or some sort of pathology. They're linked to psychosocial stress. The physical symptoms are real; they're just not due to any particular disease.

- In most people, somatization is a transient reaction to an especially stressful event, such as losing your job or getting a divorce. Or it could be due to a lower-level, but more chronic, stressor.

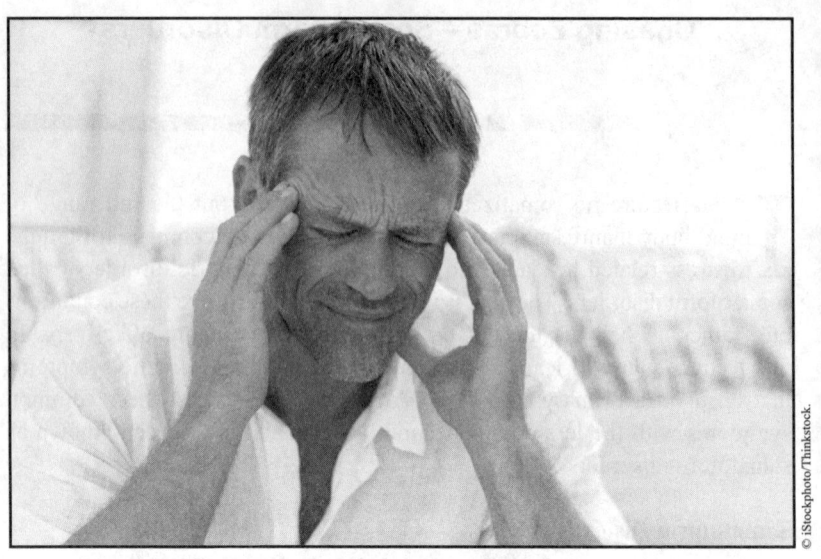

Headaches can be caused, and worsened, by stress.

The reaction consists of common physical symptoms, such as headaches, dizziness, or fatigue.

- In other patients, the process may be more persistent and disabling with no clear ties to any stressor whatsoever. It's this latter group of patients that is the most difficult for clinicians to help and understand.

- The term "psychosomatic" has a very long and storied history. It still carries some rather substantial baggage. Although it specifically professed the linkages between mind and body, "psychosomatic" was primarily limited to the practice of psychiatrist. Because of that, when the term entered into the lay public, it started to mean "it's all in your head."

- The idea of mind and body being related probably goes back as far as medicine goes back. It has been popular and unpopular at various times. Fortunately, in today's medicine, we're understanding not just that mind and body are related, but we're also understanding those biological pathways and mechanisms.

Causes of Somatic Symptoms

- Interoception is the experience of being aware of sensations inside your body, such as a feeling of hunger or pain. Proprioception is a sense of where your body is in space—of musculoskeletal awareness.

- We may, for example, all have the same amount of stomach pain, but some people, for some reasons, may at times be more sensitive interceptively than at other times. The same might be true for musculoskeletal pains, where some people have a heightened sense of proprioception.

- Under allostatic load, if you have chronic stress long enough, it starts to wear you down. Depending on where your weakest link is, that's the kind of symptom that's going to manifest (stomach ache, headache, lower back pain). This cumulative wear and tear over time, allostatic load, is going to snap that weakest link, sending you to your primary care doctor.

- Alexithymia is the inability to identify and describe emotions in the self. We might say that this is a person who has low emotional intelligence—who is detached or unplugged from his or her feelings, even though others seem to get it.

- Alexithymia is most commonly measured with the 20-item Toronto alexithymia scale. Most obviously, it's related to interpersonal conflict and relationships. It's also related to the spectrum of autistic disorders, such as Asperger's syndrome.

- In the context of somatization, it's a little bit different. Some have argued that an inability to feel your emotions predisposes someone to experience those emotions in his or her body. The theory is that a person isn't depressed; he or she has a headache, for example.

- A variant argues that it isn't about feeling emotions but about regulating emotions. If intense emotions go unregulated, they're going to take a larger toll on your body. This is very similar to the idea of allostatic load and chronic wear and tear on the individual.

- Epidemiological studies have shown that high levels of alexithymia accompany a number of different psychiatric disorders.

- About 25 to 35 percent of primary care patients have a psychiatric disorder. The most common are anxiety and depression. Both of these psychiatric disorders also have somatic symptoms. They attack or affect appetite, weight, and the ability to sleep.

- All emotions have a physiologic component; they all affect the way our bodies feel. It would make sense that if this feeling is intense enough or prolonged enough, it could have lasting effects on how our body feels.

- Sometimes it's about the sensation, but sometimes it's also about modulation or perception. Could a similar process be true in the case of emotions, where maybe we have the same feelings but we process, perceive, or modulate those feelings differently?

- Although the concept of allostatic load refers to the wear and tear from stress, we could imagine a similar system with emotions. What impact might chronic anger, fear, or depression have on an individual's body? Are we still thinking about that slow, insidious wearing down of the individual until that weakest link breaks?

- We all have habits of mind; we all take shortcuts. Sometimes those shortcuts mean that we make mountains out of molehills. We magnify or minimize things.

- We also have a tendency at times to catastrophize, which really involves looking for something to go wrong and convincing yourself that something is wrong. The treatment would be identifying that pattern and stopping those sorts of catastrophic cognitions from occurring in the first place.

- Other mechanisms could fall into the cultural or social domain. The explanatory model of illness, originally developed by Arthur Kleinman, causes us to take a step back and to think about our implicit models that we have about whatever illness that we believe we have contracted. It very much depends on the individual, but also on the family and especially on the culture.

- Our culture tells us that when we're sick, we're supposed to do certain things, such as rest and eat chicken soup. It also teaches us about particular kinds of illnesses that might be highlighted in our families or in our cultures. When a patient goes to see a primary care provider, part of what they're displaying is what they've been taught to display—their sick role or illness behavior.

- Our idioms of distress tell us that it's not okay for a man to be vulnerable or in pain or weak, for example. A little boy won't say that he's scared, but he will say that he has a stomachache instead, or an adult man won't say that he's in pain, but instead, he gets really angry because society has told him that it's okay for a man to be angry.

Recommendations for Patients with Somatization

- The first thing that health-care providers working with somatization should do is rule out whether there's some other serious disease or cause. The idea is to minimize any potential iatrogenic harm, or harm that's caused by tests, scans, or side effects from medications.

- We want to diagnose and treat things like depression or anxiety, which are quite common. We want to think about stress management interventions, such as somatic quieting, and cognitive therapies.

- We want to think about helping a patient access social supports, and mostly, we want to remove the stigma of having somatic symptoms—because we all have them. One of the best ways to do that is for medical providers to let patients know that somatic symptoms are quite common.

- Some would say that the family of psychiatric disorders known as somatoform disorders are qualitatively different from medically unexplained symptoms, but there are many similarities.

- Somatization disorder, which has to begin before age 30, endures for many years and requires frequent symptoms in multiple bodily systems, including pain, gastrointestinal, sexual, and neurologic effects. There are profound impairments in both social and occupational functioning.

- Another example is hypochondriasis, where a patient is fixated on having a particular disease despite repeated disconfirming evidence to the point of creating functional impairment. An example would be a patient who is absolutely convinced that he or she has cancer, despite multiple tests that confirm he or she actually doesn't have it.

- Fortunately, both somatization disorder and hypochondriasis can be treated with psychotherapy, but results are often mild to moderate. Therapies used include cognitive behavioral therapy and reattribution therapy, but this is certainly an area where we need to develop more effective treatments. More recently, pharmacotherapies such as SSRIs and antidepressants have been used.

Suggested Reading

Barlow, *Clinical Handbook of Psychological Disorders*.

Beck, *Cognitive Therapy*.

Bourne, *The Anxiety and Phobia Workbook*.

Satterfield, *Minding the Body*.

Questions to Consider

1. "It's all in your head" used to imply that something was imagined or made up. Now, however, we know that many stress-related symptoms are truly "in our heads." What implications does this have for personal responsibility? What about for treatment? What about for evoking empathy or support from others?

2. Although stress may not be a primary cause of most diseases, it can exacerbate most diseases and, at minimum, intensifies suffering. Why haven't pharmaceutical companies developed a "stress pill"? Why wouldn't it be beneficial to externally control the amount of stress we can feel?

Seeing the Glass Half Empty—Depression
Lecture 33

This lecture focuses on depression, the second worldwide cause of disability. In this lecture, you will learn how to define this medical disorder, and you will explore what we know about the etiology, or causes, of depression. You will also look at leading treatments for depression and emerging treatments on the horizon. Throughout this lecture, keep in mind that there is a continuum of depression and that we've all had depressive symptoms before.

Major Depression

- Sadness is usually triggered by the perception of loss, but major depression lies on the far end of the continuum. It doesn't last for hours or days, but often goes on for weeks or even months.

- Grief doesn't last just a few hours or days and might go on for extended periods of time, but with grief, there are windows of being present and being able to enjoy the relationships in your life, your job, and the things you usually enjoy. Grief comes in waves, but once depression hits, it's there to stay.

- A major depressive episode is one episode that lasts at least two weeks and may go on for a year or even more. A depressive episode means an individual has a depressed or low mood plus a loss of interest in activities for at least two weeks most of the day, nearly every day.

- An individual has to meet the criteria of five symptoms out of a list of nine. He or she has to have significant impairment and distress as a consequence of the symptoms that he or she is having. If there are no symptoms of mania or other psychiatric diagnoses, such as psychosis, then it might be called a major depressive disorder, single episode. If a person has had recurrent episodes, we would say that he or she has major depressive disorder, recurrent.

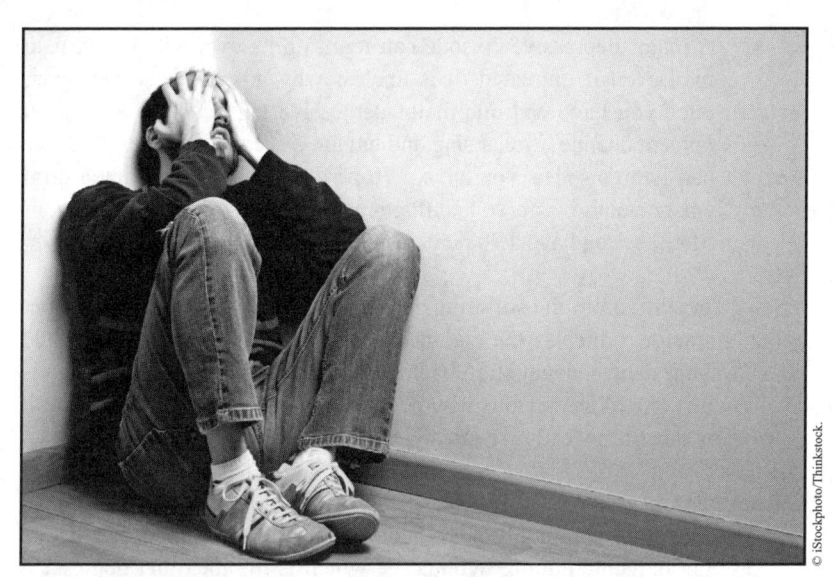

The continuum of depression ranges from having a sad mood to developing increasingly darker thoughts and feelings.

- The nine hallmark symptoms are low or depressed or irritable mood, anhedonia (inability to enjoy things that an individual usually enjoys), changes in appetite or weight, sleep changes, psychomotor agitation or retardation (a dysregulation in how an individual moves), poor concentration and poor memory, fatigue or low energy, and suicidal ideations (thoughts about hurting oneself).

- To measure disability that is caused by something like a psychiatric disease—or, for that matter, for any sort of disease—we tend to use a measure called the disability-adjusted life years (DALY), which is a statistic that was created to measure the total time lost to premature mortality plus the time living with a disability. It provides a quantitative, cumulative sum of total productive life years lost as a consequence of a disease, including diseases that might wax or wane over time.

- A major depressive episode can remit on its own within a year to two, even if untreated. It is unclear why this happens. However, once you have had one major depressive episode, you have a 50 percent chance of relapsing and having a second episode. If you've had two episodes, you have a 70 percent chance of having a third episode, and if you've had three major depressive episodes in your lifetime, you have a 90 percent chance of having a fourth.

- In addition to the suffering and morbidity, we have to worry about suicide, which is the eighth leading cause of death in the United States and accounts for about 32,000 deaths per year. Depression is just one of the reasons why people choose to commit suicide, but it is one of the leading causes.

Causes of Depression
- The most commonly held theory about the cause of depression is the biogenic aiming hypothesis, which is the idea that depression is caused by not having enough serotonin. An individual takes a selective serotonin reuptake inhibitor (SSRI), such as Prozac, Paxil, or Zoloft, and serotonin increases. Depression goes away.

- The problem with this explanation is that it's wrong. It is related to serotonin, but it takes an SSRI approximately a month or more before you start to see any sort of therapeutic effect in the individual that's taking it.

- It must be more than just the level of serotonin. It must be about the function of the neurons themselves; it must be about actual anatomical changes that are occurring within the central nervous system.

- There are, of course, new theories about what might be causing depression to occur—about the differences between two individuals that experience the same sort of life stressors and one gets depressed while the other doesn't. In this age of genomic medicine, we've been looking for genetic explanations.

- For a disease as common but as heterogeneous and complex as depression, we know there's no way we're going to find one single gene that can give us an explanation of why some people get depressed and other people don't. In fact, we believe it's a whole constellation of genes that makes a person depressed.

- There's also a theory that has to do with immune function. Depression and inflammation seem to be linked. This particular theory asserts that chronic immune activation with cytokines (chemical messengers) as mediators cause chronic inflammation and affect the central nervous system, health, and circulation.

Treatments for Depression
- Fortunately, there are a number of evidence-based treatments that are quite effective for depression. They can be used singly or in combination. Behavior therapy, cognitive behavioral therapy, and interpersonal therapy (which focuses more on relationships and life transitions) can be used, but there is also pharmacotherapy, or medications.

- Cognitive behavioral therapy for depression can be divided roughly into four stages. Stage 1 involves education about depression and data collection. In stage 2, focuses on education about behavioral activation and mood monitoring. Stage 3 moves to cognitive challenges and restructuring. Stage 4 involves addressing important social and environmental changes.

- Depression has a way of digging itself in: An individual essentially starts circling the drain and going downward, downward, downward. They can't just snap out of it, no matter how much they want to. We call this the three downward spirals of depression.

- The first spiral has to do with cognition. Depressed mood causes more negatively biased thoughts, which cause a person to be more depressed, which causes them to think more negatively, which causes them to be more depressed, and so on.

- With the second downward spiral, depressed mood causes people to have less interest, less enjoyment, and less energy, so it causes people to be less active, which makes them more depressed, which makes them less active, which makes them more depressed, and so on.

- The last downward spiral has to do with social contacts. Depressed mood lowers social contacts. People don't enjoy the support, relationships, or activities anymore. They often become hypersensitive to rejection or very self-conscious. They don't want to be around other people. Depressed mood lowers social contacts, which makes them more depressed, which lowers social contacts, which makes them more depressed, and so on.

- There are also medications for depression. There are multiple classes of drugs, but the most commonly used are the selective serotonin reuptake inhibitors (SSRIs). These particular drugs take about four to six weeks to work. Fortunately, they have very few side effects, and they're fairly safe in overdose compared to other antidepressants.

- There are also supplements for depression, such as Saint-John's-wort or *Hypericum perforatum*, which is a yellow flowering herb indigenous to Europe that is considered a natural herbal treatment for depression. However, there is a recent finding that Saint-John's-wort increases liver metabolism and actually flushes other drugs that you might be taking out of your system.

- A different adjunctive agent is called S-adenosylmethionine (SAMe), which is a naturally occurring molecule that appears to be an effective and well-tolerated adjunctive treatment for depression. It's not used as a monotherapy but as an adjunctive therapy.

- Electroconvulsive therapy (ECT), which is sometimes called shock therapy, has been around for about 100 years. The idea is that you electrically and purposefully induce a seizure in a depressed person in order to derive some sort of therapeutic benefit. ECT is only used in cases of severe treatment-resistant depression, and it's much more humane than it was in the past. There is good evidence that ECT works, but relapse tends to happen in six months.

- A combination of cognitive therapy and medications seems to be your best bet for depression. The medications will take four to six weeks to work, and cognitive therapy takes several weeks to work. The difference comes in relapse rates, which tend to be lower for cognitive therapy.

- The other alternative is aerobic exercise, which increases brain-derived neurotrophic factors. In fact, there are a number of randomized, controlled trials showing that exercise is effective in lowering depression even if the effects are minimal.

- There are a number of interesting emerging treatments, such as vagus nerve stimulation or transcranial magnetic stimulation, which uses a metal coil to release electromagnetic impulses. These seem to work. The effects are less effective than ECT, but certainly a little bit less traumatic.

Suggested Reading

Barlow, *Clinical Handbook of Psychological Disorders*.

Beck, *Cognitive Therapy*.

Burns, *Feeling Good*.

Greenberger and Padesky, *Mind over Mood*.

Satterfield, *Minding the Body*.

Solomon, *The Noonday Demon*.

Thompson, *The Beast*.

Questions to Consider

1. Prevalence rates for major depression have been slowly rising over the past several decades—particularly in Western countries. What might explain this troubling finding? Recall that depression is currently the top cause of disability in adults 15 to 44 years old worldwide. What's going on, and what can be done about it?

2. What are the positive and negative ramifications of the increasingly accepted biological model of depression? If technology eventually creates more effective antidepressant medication, is there something that we will lose by ignoring other interventions?

Silencing the Scream—Understanding Anxiety
Lecture 34

In this lecture, you will learn about the largest and most common family of psychiatric disorders: the anxiety disorders. You will use the biopsychosocial model to help explain cause, treatment, and prevention. You will also learn what fear and anxiety are, and you will discover the important functions that they sometimes serve. In addition, you will be introduced to the different members within the family of anxiety disorders, such as simple phobias, obsessive-compulsive disorder, post-traumatic stress disorder, social anxiety, and panic disorder. Finally, you will learn about pharmacologic interventions and cognitive therapy.

Anxiety Disorders

- Anxiety and anxiety disorders lie on the same continuum as depression, with anxiety disorders at one end, and all of us have experienced some level of fear or anxiety. Fear and anxiety are normal psychological and physiologic responses to danger.

- In general, fear is conceptualized as an emotional and physiological response to a threat. Fear is a universal emotion; it is primal. It serves an important function: to help us identify a threat and hopefully to survive.

- Anxiety is influenced by culture, cognition, personality, and any number of other internal factors. Anxiety can trigger fear, and fear can result in lingering anxiety.

- Fear and anxiety are universal emotions that have a purpose, but at some point, their functionality begins to decrease. They become false alarms or false triggers. They no longer seem to be helpful.

- Anxiety disorders refer to a heterogeneous group of syndromes characterized by abnormally increased sensitivity to fearful stimuli, an inappropriately intense experience of fear or anxiety, or an inappropriately extreme action based on the fear or anxiety that you just had.

- Essentially, there's a wide range of normal fears in the population. There are large cultural differences in what's considered normal, but we have a pretty good idea in terms of the sensitivity of that trigger—the magnitude and duration of a response—that pushes an individual into the category of having an anxiety disorder. The diagnosis of anxiety disorder is based primarily on the degree of interference with normal function at work or in your social life.

- A little bit of anxiety is actually a good thing; it gives you energy and arousal. In fact, a little bit of anxiety or fear might even improve your performance. The Yerkes-Dodson curve plots anxiety level on one axis and performance on another axis.

- When you have zero anxiety, performance tends to be low. When you have moderate anxiety, performance tends to be high. With high anxiety, performance drops back down. This forms a classic inverted-U shape.

- Stress and anxiety tend to overlap, both psychologically as well as physiologically. Given that anxiety is often a more diffuse, longer-lasting state, how is it different from what we've been calling chronic stress? It might be helpful to think about anxiety as being a subcomponent or a particular kind of emotional response to stress.

- For anxiety disorders, though, the anxiety has gotten so extreme that it has taken on a life of its own. The disorder becomes a mental illness. Although it isn't always the case, many anxiety disorders can start with chronic stress and be exacerbated by chronic stress.

Diagnostic Classifications of Anxiety Disorders
- The category of anxiety disorders is the largest family of psychiatric disorders. One in four people will have an anxiety disorder at some point in their lifetime. Fortunately, nearly all of the anxiety disorders are imminently treatable.

- Simple phobias include fear of heights, fear of closed spaces, and arachnophobia (fear of spiders). We all have fears, but someone who would meet criteria for a phobia has functional impairment as a consequence of their fear. They're not able to work or fly, for example, because of their fear.

- What used to be called social phobia is now called social anxiety disorder (SAD). This is not just shyness amplified. People who have social anxiety disorder have an intense fear of being in public—and, particularly, being observed in public. Sometimes it's a generalized sense of not knowing what to say or do or feeling self-conscious while other times it's much more specific and localized.

- Panic disorder is another member of this family. Most people have at least one panic attack at some point in their life. It is a sudden physiologic rush of intense fear (fight-or-flight response). Often, people don't have a second attack, but if they do, or if they become preoccupied with having a future attack, they might meet criteria for panic disorder.

- People who have generalized anxiety disorder (GAD) are chronic worrywarts. Of course, all of us worry from time to time, but people with GAD spend more than 50 percent of their time worrying. In fact, they have worried so much that they start to have a lot of somatic, or bodily, symptoms that are caused by their chronic worry.

- As its name implies, there are two pieces to obsessive-compulsive disorder (OCD): unwanted, intrusive thoughts called obsessions; and an irresistible impulse to do something, which are the compulsions. The problem with OCD is that compulsive behavior only works in the short term, and they are trapped in a cycle of performing a task over and over.

- Post-traumatic stress disorder (PTSD) is essentially an ongoing, sometimes chronic response after an individual is exposed to a traumatic life event.

The Biology of Anxiety Disorders

- The risk for developing anxiety disorders has a genetic component. In fact, most estimates of twin studies show that the heritability is between 20 and 30 percent. However, this also means that 70 to 80 percent of what explains who gets an anxiety disorder doesn't have to do with genetics.

- Psychosocial variables might also help us understand why a person develops an anxiety disorder. Maybe some people are more genetically vulnerable. Then, when they have that keystone event that occurs, they're off and running with a new anxiety disorder.

- Epigenetics involves turning genetic switches on or off. This does not involve actually changing the genome or the DNA, but activating or inactivating particular genes that might be related to anxiety.

- Much of fear is based in the amygdala. Chronic activation of the amygdala, which is what happens with post-traumatic stress disorder, often causes hippocampal shrinkage, which could affect memories.

- Across all of the anxiety disorders, there is a hyperreactivity to fearful stimuli and an underregulation of emotion. Essentially, an individual's trigger has become too sensitive. The magnitude of the response he or she has, once triggered, is much too high. The response, once it's turned on, lasts too long.

- This exaggerated trigger, response, and duration implies involvement of sensory processing in the thalamus, the amygdala, and the hypothalamus as well as their bidirectional connections with the frontal lobes and the prefrontal cortex.

- Most of us, when we feel fear or anxiety, can talk ourselves back from having an exaggerated anxiety response. That's very difficult to do in the case of anxiety disorders.

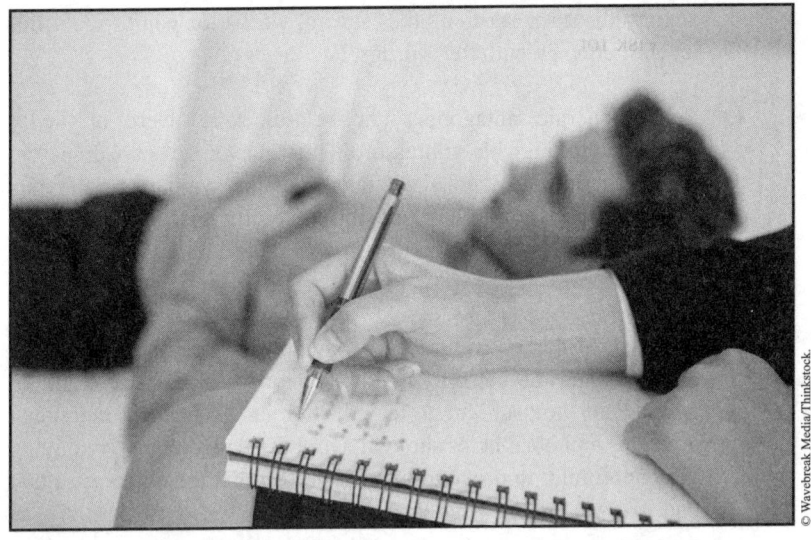

There are a number of different types of therapies that are used to treat anxiety disorders.

Pharmacotherapies and Psychotherapies

- The pharmacotherapies for anxiety disorders are benzodiazepines, which are sometimes called tranquilizers, sedatives, or hypnotics. These are drugs like Xanax, Ativan, or Valium. These drugs are remarkably effective in reducing excitability in the amygdala. They seem to decrease activation of the fear circuit.

- These sorts of drugs are often prescribed for panic disorder, but they shouldn't be used as frontline treatments. They can provide very rapid benefits, but the long-term risk is that the individual becomes dependent on or even addicted to the drug. There are also a number of side effects, including drowsiness and loss of concentration.

- Frontline treatments for panic disorder and some of the other anxiety disorders are antidepressants, which affect cortical processes that stimulate fear circuitry. Antidepressants are often used in longer-term management of panic disorder and generalized anxiety disorder. It often takes several weeks for you to see a full level of efficacy with these drugs.

- Beta-adrenergic antagonists, or beta-blockers, were originally developed for high blood pressure. They antagonize beta-adrenergic receptors, turning down the intensity of the sympathetic nervous system response. The caveat with these drugs is if you take too high of a dose, your blood pressure actually bottoms out and you will faint.

- There are many cognitive behavioral therapies for anxiety disorders. On the behavioral side, some of the components might include an exposure to a feared stimulus. When an individual develops a phobia, he or she will avoid the feared object, removing the opportunity to prove to him- or herself that the object isn't that bad. We want to diminish this avoidance.

- Cognitive components deal with challenging catastrophic cognitions. When we are afraid, we have all sorts of magnified thoughts about the severity of the danger that we're in. We probably want to pull those thoughts back down to something that's a little bit smaller.

- We often see a mix of behavioral and cognitive strategies, things that help us to do what's called reality testing. Are you magnifying or minimizing the real danger of a situation?

- Instead of sympathetic activation, you want to learn ways to activate your parasympathetic nervous system, which often requires some level of focused concentration, a quiet environment, and a passive, noncompetitive, unambitious attitude. This might include meditation, progressive muscle relaxation, or guided imagery.

Suggested Reading

Barlow, *Clinical Handbook of Psychological Disorders.*

Beck, *Cognitive Therapy.*

Bourne, *The Anxiety and Phobia Workbook.*

Davis, Eshelman, and McKay, *The Relaxation and Stress Reduction Wookbook.*

Greenberger and Padesky, *Mind over Mood.*

Satterfield, *Minding the Body.*

Questions to Consider

1. Is an individual's set point for anxiety a product of nature or nurture? How could you test this, and why would it matter? Use what you know about epigenetics, social supports, and the emergence of modern stressors.

2. Should medicine attempt to even out the level of anxiety that all people feel so that none are more or less anxious than others in a given social context? Why would variability be a good thing?

Lingering Wounds—Trauma, Resilience, Growth
Lecture 35

This lecture focuses a little more deeply on a specific anxiety disorder: post-traumatic stress disorder. The Substance Abuse and Mental Health Services Administration notes that individual trauma results from an event, a series of events, or a set of circumstances that is experienced by an individual as physically or emotionally harmful or threatening and that has lasting adverse effects on the individual's functioning and physical, social, emotional, and spiritual well-being. In this lecture, you will learn about the negative effects of post-traumatic stress disorder. You will also learn about post-traumatic growth, which is the possibility of being resilient and becoming stronger after a trauma occurs.

Trauma Disorders

- Traumatic events overwhelm the usual methods of coping that give people a sense of control, connection, and meaning. Traumatic events include sexual assault or rape, combat, car accidents, and even vicarious traumatic experiences. In other words, you can observe a trauma happening to another person and be traumatized yourself and potentially even develop post-traumatic stress disorder.

- Unfortunately—but with the exception of sexual molestation, sexual assault, and rape—trauma is much more likely to happen to a man than to a woman.

- With traumas, there's often a spectrum of responses. We expect anyone that undergoes a trauma to be affected by that trauma. Sleeplessness, rumination, and losing one's temper or having mood swings are all normal and expected responses to trauma, but we want to place these different disorders on a continuum.

- The DSM-IV, the Diagnostic and Statistical Manual of Mental Disorders, put out by the American Psychiatric Association, creates a list of what they call trauma-related disorders—from the least severe to the most severe.

- In the least severe category, they list bereavement. Not that bereavement is considered a psychiatric disorder, at least not yet, but bereavement is something that can last up to a full year. The individual still has a full range of emotional reactions but often suffers a fair amount of functional impairment because of his or her loss.

- The next trauma-related disorder is the family of adjustment disorders. We all have reactions to trauma, but an adjustment disorder is something that's more intense and lasts longer than you might expect given the stressor or the trauma that has happened. This might include an anxiety reaction, depression or anger; apathy or detachment; or somatic symptoms. It usually doesn't last more than six months after the trauma occurs or after the chronic stressor or other trigger has ended.

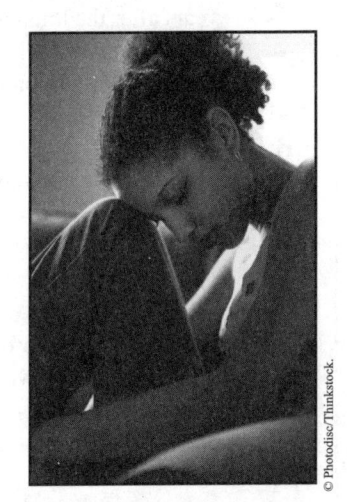

Traumatic events overwhelm the usual methods of coping.

- Acute stress disorder lasts up to four weeks after a trauma occurs. Essentially, most researchers and clinicians think about acute stress disorder as the prodrome, or precursor, for developing full-blown post-traumatic stress disorder (PTSD).

- At the end of the spectrum for trauma-related disorder is PTSD, for which the hallmark symptom is reexperiencing the trauma over and over again through flashbacks or nightmares. There is also the characteristic anxious avoidance of things that might remind them of the trauma. PTSD can last for years.

- Curiously, and we don't understand why, PTSD doesn't always immediately follow a trauma. Sometimes it can actually occur years after the trauma has occurred. Somehow that trauma had been suppressed, but when it starts to resurface, the individual starts experiencing symptoms of post-traumatic stress disorder.

Criteria of PTSD
- In the DSM-IV, which was published in 1994, the criteria of post-traumatic stress disorder include an exposure to a traumatic event with actual or threatened death or serious injury and a response involving intense fear, helplessness, or horror.

- Other criteria, according to the DSM-IV, include reexperiencing the traumatic event—which is referring to flashbacks and nightmares—and persistent avoidance of stimuli that are associated with the event. There are a number of fear-based memories that are put down when a person is traumatized, including a general numbing of responsiveness and emotions and symptoms of increased arousal.

- Symptoms have to last for at least one month; otherwise, the individual might be diagnosed with acute stress disorder, which is a precursor, or prodrome, that can't last for more than four weeks. In addition, there is significant stress or impairment in social, occupational, or other functioning.

Risk Factors for PTSD
- Even though PTSD is common, it certainly doesn't happen to everyone—in fact, not to most people—who have had a trauma. The biggest single predictor is the severity of the trauma itself. Another predictor is a history of prior traumatization.

- Gender is also a risk factor. For reasons that we don't fully understand, in general, even though traumas are more likely to happen to men, PTSD is more likely to happen to women.

- Having a prior mood or anxiety disorder is a risk factor, as is having a family history—for example, a parent or sibling who has had a mood or anxiety disorder. In addition, the onset of PTSD is related to having low education, although we don't understand the mechanisms.

- Even though we have a list of DSM criteria of PTSD and the kinds of suffering it causes, PTSD often pushes people who have it to cope in ways that are maladaptive. One of the most common ways is through alcohol and drug use. Other associated features are often aggression or violence, particularly in men. We may see suicidal ideation or even suicide attempts.

- In addition, we might see dissociation, where things seem very unreal. There might be distancing from friends and family, pulling away from social supports, problems at work, marital problem, or even homelessness.

- There are a number of psychobiological findings with post-traumatic stress disorder. We see increased physiologic responses to trauma-related cues, meaning that anything that reminds them of the trauma is met with a rapid and intense fight-or-flight response. We see increased heart-rate responses to startling noises. We see increased reactivity to adrenergic stimulation. For unclear reasons, we see smaller hippocampal volume.

- Interestingly, we see decreased sleep efficiency. It's difficult to fall asleep and stay asleep, but once individuals with PTSD are asleep, they spend more time in REM sleep, presumably having nightmares.

- Lastly, we see higher levels of circulating catecholamines in the bloodstream basically throughout the entire day. Those catecholamines are epinephrine and norepinephrine.

Pharmacotherapies
- There are pharmacotherapies that can be helpful for PTSD, but there aren't any that are especially so. Randomized, controlled trials looking at different medications versus placebos work in about half of the studies and don't work in about half of the studies.

- In general, the most positive effects come from SSRIs, such as Zoloft and Paxil. These tended to have the best results, but they still only helped about half to two-thirds of the individuals.

- Sometimes providers will turn to benzodiazepines, including Xanax, Klonopin, Alprazolam, or Clonazepam, to help patients with post-traumatic stress disorder. For chronic PTSD, the same medications have been tried. They help lower anxiety levels, but they don't really help with the core symptoms of post-traumatic stress disorder.

- Beta-blockers have also been used to treat post-traumatic stress disorder as a way to pull down the sympathetic nervous system. The results that come from studies examining the effects of beta-blockers need to be replicated, however.

- Most of us won't develop post-traumatic stress disorder even though we might experience bereavement or an incurable illness or some sort of irreparable psychological or physical damage. We can use problem-focused coping and emotion-focused coping to help cope with these sorts of events.

- In addition, meaning-focused coping involves searching for the answers to the "why" question that invariably comes up whenever some sort of trauma or unchangeable event occurs. This type of coping could be very important for people who experience a traumatic event.

- Post-traumatic growth does happen, but it's not definite. We're not sure how to predict it, promote it, or control it. Remember that cognitive restructuring and managing anger are important, and forgiveness begins with a decision.

- It is important to find meaning even in suffering, and often, altruism can give us that meaning. There are practical ways that we can promote resilience and growth in others. We can learn to ask about and reinforce strengths. We can bear witness or listen as someone shares his or her traumatic story. We can use our power as a surrogate or place of refuge.

Suggested Reading

Barlow, *Clinical Handbook of Psychological Disorders.*

Beck, *Cognitive Therapy.*

Bourne, *The Anxiety and Phobia Workbook.*

Chodron, *When Things Fall Apart.*

Frankl, *Man's Search for Meaning.*

Hayes, *Get Out of Your Mind and Into Your Life.*

Reivich and Shatte, *The Resilience Factor.*

Rothbaum, Foa, and Hembree, *Reclaiming Your Life from a Traumatic Experience.*

Satterfield, *A Cognitive-Behavioral Approach to the Beginning of the End of Life: Minding the Body.* New York: Oxford University Press, 2008.

———, *Minding the Body.*

Questions to Consider

1. If rumination amplifies negative emotions and intensifies suffering, why would telling a traumatic story over and over again with a therapist be helpful? Why doesn't this make people with post-traumatic stress disorder worse?

2. What exactly does it mean to say that someone is "healed" after a trauma? Why do some wounds heal while others never do?

Tomorrow's Biopsychosocial Medicine
Lecture 36

This final lecture will attempt to look into the near future to anticipate changes to health and health care that might arise from an increased attention to the biopsychosocial factors. Specifically, in this lecture, you will learn about upcoming changes in medical care and health education. You will also learn about the exciting promises of medicine and health for the future. Hopefully, this course has inspired you to try something new—meditation, exercise, cognitive therapy, journaling, or even mood-induction exercises.

The Three Ts of Health Transformation: Technology

- It is time to change the way medicine is taught and practiced. A confluence of factors is pushing us toward change, including out-of-control health-care costs that aren't accompanied by an increase in quality, a dysfunctional health-care and payment reimbursement system, increasingly disturbing data on health and health-care disparities, and the increasing diversity and aging of our population.

- Another problem is the condition of our health-care providers. There are unprecedented rates of burnout and compassion fatigue, and the number of medical errors that occur is appalling. A transformation is going to occur through the three Ts of health transformation: technology, touch, and teaching.

- In Eric Topol's fascinating and somewhat provocative book, *The Creative Destruction of Medicine*, he describes how the digital revolution is irreversibly changing the face of medicine—so much that it will essentially destroy the old medical models of the past and supplant them with something entirely different.

- There needs to be a world-changing, irreversible revolution in the ways that information is stored and retrieved. Medical school is no longer about memorizing vast amounts of information or becoming a walking medical encyclopedia. It's about how to effectively and efficiently search for information, evaluate that information, and translate it into clinical care—a process that starts with what is now called medical informatics and ends with evidence-based medicine and translational science. All of this storage and retrieval capacity causes all sorts of new challenges.

- We've also changed the ways that we communicate. There are approximately 6 billion cell phones in use around the world, and 300 billion email messages are sent every day. Email and texting are increasingly common ways for medical teams to communicate with one another and for patients and their medical team to communicate with one another.

- There's also the electronic health record, which is mostly stored on secure servers now but will probably live in the cloud at some point in the near future. It promises to better coordinate our health care and provide the most comprehensive, up-to-date information regarding our health and health-care needs (with risks to privacy and other concerns, of course).

- But technology is not just about the digital revolution; it's also about science and biomedical science. Personalized medicine is the very real possibility of being able to subtype an individual or a disease so that we can pick out precisely the right medication that might work for him or her, which is what we're already doing for patients with HIV or cancer.

- With the help of genomics, we might be able to identify the risk that an individual might have for developing chronic diseases in the future so that we can start preventive interventions early.

- Just 20 years ago, we didn't have MRIs; now we have PET scans, SPECT scans, fMRIs, DEXA scans, and so on. This list of high-tech tools and machines in hospitals will continue to grow.

- It's not just about high-tech gadgets; it's also about home health monitoring, with both external and implanted devices that we will manage ourselves. There are now pill bottles that will call your doctor if you forget to take your medicine. There are accelerometers that count your steps as you walk throughout the day and similar devices that monitor your quality of sleep.

- Soon, we may have nanorobots that are able to image the inside of our blood vessels as an early intervention to prevent or treat cardiovascular disease. It's a very different medical world now, and it's going to get a lot stranger.

The Three Ts of Health Transformation: Touch

- In the face of all of this technology, some fear that we might lose the touch, or the relationships, referring to the classic concept of good bedside manner—or, in the medical education field, this is described as professionalism, presence, or empathy.

- Research shows that this isn't just a nice thing to do; in fact, medical outcomes are improved when patients feel connected to their medical providers. In addition, medical providers feel less burned out when they're connected to their patients.

- We're experiencing resistance from what can be dehumanizing technology, but care that can be high tech can still be high touch. There will always be a range of providers with different bedside manners, but a movement is underway to teach medicine through service.

- Rather than learning about patients as collections of organs, students will learn about patients as people first, by learning to work with them as medical assistants. In the medicine of tomorrow, we need to remember that it will be less exclusively focused on the provider or even the medical team. Medicine will include you, your family, potentially your friends, and even your community.

- If we think broadly and consider ourselves citizens of the globe, we need to remember to build awareness about global health conditions and the interconnectedness of health for all people. This would include thinking about ways to finally eradicate HIV. We need to keep our interconnectedness to be able to face any global pandemics, including diseases such as SARS or H1N1.

The Three Ts of Health Transformation: Teaching

- The third T stands for "teaching," and in this case, we're referring to teaching health professionals. Fortunately, there have been a number of important changes to medical education in just the past few years.

- First, there are now new pre-medical requirements. In a few years, any medical student who wants to apply to medical school will need to have taken a class, at least on an introductory level, of psychology and/or sociology or anthropology.

- Starting in 2015, on the new Medical College Admission Test (MCAT), which every student has to take to get into medical school, nearly half of all the core concepts are from the social and behavioral sciences.

- In 2011, the Association of American Medical Colleges released standards or objectives for behavioral and social science education. Hopefully, the first comprehensive, high-level biopsychosocial textbook is going to be released under the auspices of the American Psychosomatic Society in just a few years.

- It's not just about changes in content; it's also about changes in pedagogy, or the way that we teach. It's about curricular innovations. Teaching curricula are moving to learning curricula. We're using more case-based teaching so that it's easier to translate science into clinical practice.

- There are a number of other important innovations, such as a new medical school in Taiwan that has based their entire curriculum around compassion. Rather than starting medical school by dissecting an anonymous cadaver, students actually learn who their cadaver is and meet the family. They build a relationship with them. Eventually, they attend the services for the cremation or burial of the cadaver—the loved one of the family.

- In New York City, to prevent residents from getting burned out, the residents are able to go with their patients back to their home to do house calls so that they can build a more professional, or personal, relationship.

- At the Georgetown University School of Medicine, Adviad Haramati is leading the charge to teach mindfulness to medical students. It has been so incredibly popular that both the School of Business and the Law Center have started teaching mindfulness.

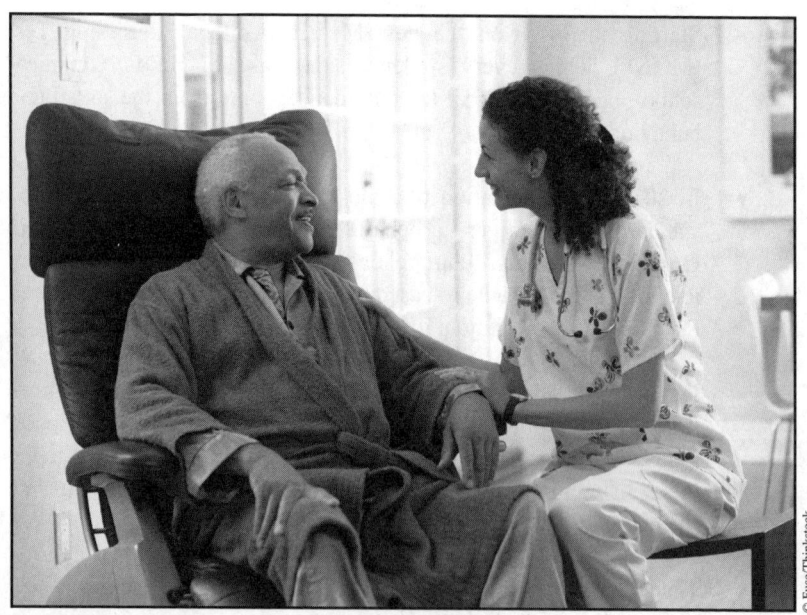

Medical outcomes are improved when patients feel connected to their medical providers.

- Knowing what or how your doctor has been trained helps you know what to expect. Knowing what to expect, when to speak up, and what sorts of questions to ask are all critical skills for all patients to develop.

Health Care of the Future
- Health-care teams of the future will be interdisciplinary—they'll have shared duties. There will be more nonphysicians. Physicians and medical teams will be more sophisticated in thinking about psychology, behavioral factors, and social factors. This will be due to changes in training, patient empowerment, electronic medical records, and information technology solutions.

- Hopefully, we'll have a new breed of psychologist and physician, where each knows more about the other discipline. We'll also have patients, families, and communities all included as part of the team.

- What does this future mean for you? Initially, it means that there are going to be more providers and a larger health-care team, so there will be more people to get to know and more coordination that is needed. There will be more empowerment for you, but there will also be more responsibility.

- What can you do to help make these changes happen? Start your own biopsychosocial assessment. Use the various assessment tools that are available to identify your strengths, challenges, and opportunities.

- In addition, consider having an annual biopsychosocial checkup. If your regular health-care provider is not able to do this, consider a behavioral psychologist or someone trained in mind-body medicine.

Suggested Reading

Association of American Medical Colleges, *Behavioral and Social Science Foundations for Future Physicians*.

Institute of Medicine, *Behavioral and Social Sciences in Medical School Curricula*.

Schattner, "The Silent Dimension."

Schimpff, *The Future of Medicine*.

Spector, "Germs Are Us."

Topol, *The Creative Destruction of Medicine*.

Questions to Consider

1. Is it possible for medicine in the future to be both high tech and high touch? Technology dollars and scientific research will push high tech, but what will promote high touch?

2. Do you agree that we have reached a tipping point in regard to the meaningful integration of the biopsychosocial model in health care? If so, what will this mean on a practical level? If not, what will it take to finally make integration happen?

Bibliography

Abbas, A., A. Lichtman, and S. Pillai. *Basic Immunology: Functions and Disorders of the Immune System*. Philadelphia, PA: Elsevier, 2012.

Adler, N. E., and J. Stewart. "Health Disparities across the Lifespan: Meaning, Methods, and Mechanisms." *Annals of the New York Academy of Sciences* 1186 (2010): 5–23.

American Dietetic Association. *Complete Food and Nutrition Guide*. 3rd ed. Hoboken, NJ: Wiley Press, 2006.

American Psychosomatic Society. Organizational website with educational materials for a range of somatic conditions. Available at www.psychosomatic.org. Last accessed 1/3/2013.

Ariely, D. *Predictably Irrational: The Hidden Forces That Shape Our Decisions*. New York: Harper Collins, 2008.

Association of American Medical Colleges. *Behavioral and Social Science Foundations for Future Physicians*. Washington, DC: Association of American Medical Colleges, 2011.

Barlow, D. H. *Clinical Handbook of Psychological Disorders*. 3rd ed. New York: Guilford Press, 2001.

Bath, J., G. Bohin, C. Jone, and E. Scarle. *Cardiac Rehabilitation: A Workbook for Group Programs*. New York: Wiley, 2009.

Baumeister, R. F., and J. Tierney. *Willpower: Rediscovering the Greatest Human Strength*. New York: Penguin Books, 2011.

Beck, A. T. *Prisoners of Hate: The Cognitive Basis of Anger, Hostility, and Violence*. New York: Harper Collins, 1999.

Beck, J. S. *Cognitive Therapy: Basics and Beyond.* New York: Guilford, 1995.

Becker, C. M., M. A. Glascoff, and W. M. Felts. "Salutogenesis 30 Years Later: Where Do We Go from Here?" *International Electronic Journal of Health Education* 13 (2010): 25–32.

Benson, H., and M. Z. Klipper. *The Relaxation Response.* New York: Harper Torch, 1976.

Blessing, B., and I. Gibbons. "Autonomic Nervous System." *Scholarpedia* 3, no.7 (2008): 2787. Accessed at http://www.scholarpedia.org/article/Autonomic_nervous_system on 1/3/2013.

Bourne, E. J. *The Anxiety and Phobia Workbook.* 3rd ed. San Francisco, CA: New Harbinger Press, 2000.

Breedlove, S. M., N. V. Watson, and M. R. Rosenzsweig. *Biological Psychology: An Introduction to Behavioral, Cognitive, and Clinical Neuroscience.* 6th ed. Sunderland, MA: Sinauer Associates Press, 2005.

Bronfenbrenner, U. *The Ecology of Human Development: Experiments by Nature and Design.* Cambridge, MA: Harvard University Press, 1979.

Brooks, D. *The Social Animal: The Hidden Sources of Love, Character, and Achievement.* New York: Random House, 2011.

Brownell, K. D., R. Kersh, D. D. Ludwig, R. C. Post, R. M. Puhl, M. B. Schwartz, and W. C. Willett. "Personal Responsibility and Obesity: A Constructive Approach to a Controversial Issue." *Health Affairs* 29, no. 3 (March 2010): 378–386.

Burns, D. D. *Feeling Good: The New Mood Therapy.* New York: Signet, 1980.

Caudill-Slosberg, M. *Managing Pain Before It Manages You.* New York: Guilford Publications, 2001.

Chodron, P. *When Things Fall Apart: Heart Advice for Difficult Times*. New ed. Boston, MA: Shambhala Publications, Inc., 2000.

Covey, S. R. *The 7 Habits of Highly Effective People*. 15th ed. New York: Free Press, 2004.

Cox, T., A. Griffiths, and E. Rial-Gonzalez. *Research on Work-Related Stress*. Luxembourg: Office for Official Publication of the European Communities, 2000. https://osha.europa.eu/en/publications/reports/203.

Damasio, A. *Looking for Spinoza: Joy, Sorrow, and the Feeling Brain*. Orlando, FL: Harcourt Press, 2003.

Davidson, R. J., et al. "Alterations in Brain and Immune Function Produced by Mindfulness Meditation." *Psychosomatic Medicine* 65 (2003): 564-570.

Davis, M., E. R. Eshelman, and M. McKay. *The Relaxation and Stress Reduction Wookbook*. 5th ed. San Francisco, CA: New Harbinger, 2000.

Digman, J. M. "Personality Structure: Emergence of the Five-Factor Model." *Annual Review of Psychology* 41 (1990): 417–440.

Dossey, L. *Prayer Is Good Medicine: How to Reap the Healing Benefits of Prayer*. San Francisco: Harper, 1997.

Duhigg, C. *The Power of Habit: Why We Do What We Do in Life and Business*. New York: Random House, 2012.

Duncan, J. *How Intelligence Happens*. New Haven, CT: Yale University Press, 2010.

Dunn, A. L., R. E. Andersen, and J. M. Jakicic. "Lifestyle Physical Activity Interventions: History, Short- and Long-Term Effects, and Recommendations." *American Journal of Preventative Medicine* 15, no. 4 (1998): 398–412.

Ekman, P. *Emotions Revealed: Recognizing Faces and Feelings to Improve Communication and Emotional Life*. New York: Times Books, 2003.

Engel, G. L. "The Clinical Application of the Biopsychosocial Model." *American Journal of Psychiatry* 137 (1980): 535–544.

———. "The Need for a New Medical Model: A Challenge for Biomedicine." *Science* 196 (1977): 129–136.

Engel, P. A. "George L. Engel, M.D., 1913–1999: Remembering His Life and Work; Rediscovering His Soul. *Psychosomatics* 42 (2001): 94–99.

Enright, R. D. *Forgiveness Is a Choice: A Step-by-Step Process for Resolving Anger and Restoring Hope*. Washington, DC: American Psychological Association, 2001.

Estabrook, P. A., R. E. Glasgow, and D. A. Dzewaltowski. "Physical Activity Promotion through Primary Care." *Journal of the American Medical Association* 289, no. 22 (2003): 2913–2916.

Fanning, P., and J. T. O'Neill. *The Addiction Workbook*. San Francisco: New Harbinger Press, 1996.

Folkman, S., and J. T. Moskowitz. "Coping: Pitfalls and Promises." *Annual Review of Psychology* 55 (2004): 745–74.

Frankl, V. *Man's Search for Meaning: An Introduction to Logotherapy*. Boston, MA: Beacon Press, 1959.

Gardner, C. D., A. Kiazand, S. Alhassan, et al. "Comparison of the Atkins, Zone, Ornish, and LEARN Diets for Change in Weight and Related Risk Factors among Overweight Premenopausal Women: The A TO Z Weight Loss Study: A Randomized Trial." *Journal of the American Medical Association* 297, no. 9 (2007): 969–977.

Gardner, D., and D. Shoback. *Greenspan's Basic and Clinical Endocrinology*. 9th ed. New York: McGraw-Hill, 2011.

Geronimus, A. T., M. Hicken, D. Keene, and J. Bound. "'Weathering' and Age Patterns of Allostatic Load Scores among Blacks and Whites in the United States." *American Journal of Public Health* 96, no. 5 (2006): 826–833.

Goleman, D. *Emotional Intelligence*. New York: Bantam, 1995.

Gottman, J. M., and N. Silver. *The 7 Principles for Making Marriage Work*. New York: Three Rivers Press, 2000.

Greenberger, D., and C. A. Padesky. *Mind over Mood: A Cognitive Therapy Treatment Manual for Clients*. New York: Guilford, 1995.

Hayes, S. *Get Out of Your Mind and Into Your Life: The New Acceptance and Commitment Therapy*. Oakland, CA: New Harbinger Publications, Inc., 2005.

Helms, J. E. "Black and White Racial Identity: Theory, Research, and Practice." *Contributions in Afro-American and African Studies*. No. 129. New York: Greenwood Press, 1990.

Hendrix, H. *Getting the Love You Want: A Guide for Couples*. 20th ed. New York: Holt Paperbacks, 2008.

Hurley, D. "Can You Make Yourself Smarter?" *The New York Times*. April 18, 2012.

Institute of Medicine. *Behavioral and Social Sciences in Medical School Curricula*. Washington, DC: National Academies Press, 2004.

———. *Cancer Care for the Whole Patient*. Washington, DC: National Academies Press, 2007.

———. *Unequal Treatment: Confronting Racial and Ethnic Disparities in Health Care*. Washington, DC: National Academies Press, 2002.

Jacobs, G. D. *Say Goodnight to Insomnia*. New York: Holt, 1998.

Johnson, S. *Mind Wide Open: Your Brain and the Neuroscience of Everyday Life*. New York: Scribner Press, 2004.

Kabat-Zinn, J. *Full Catastrophe Living: Using the Wisdom of Your Body and Mind to Face Stress, Pain, and Illness*. New York: Bantam Dell, 1990.

Kessler, D. *The End of Overeating: Taking Control of the Insatiable American Appetite*. New York: Rodale, Inc., 2009.

King, N., and R. Straus, et al. *The Social Medicine Reader*. 2nd ed. Vols. 1–3. Durham, NC: Duke University Press, 2005.

Koenig, H., D. King, and V. B. Carson. *Handbook of Religion and Health*. New York: Oxford University Press, 2012.

Kringelbach, M. L., and K. C. Berridge. *Pleasures of the Brain*. New York: Oxford University Press, 2010.

Larsen, R., and D. Buss. *Personality Psychology: Domains of Knowledge about Human Nature*. New York: McGraw-Hill, 2009.

Lazarus, R. S., and S. Folkman. *Stress, Appraisal, and Coping*. New York: Springer, 1984.

Lehrer, P. M., R. L. Woolfolk, and W. E. Sime. *Principles and Practice of Stress Management*. 3rd ed. New York: Guilford Press, 2007.

Luskin, F. *Forgive for Good: A Proven Prescription for Health and Happiness*. New York: HarperOne, 2003.

Macarthur Foundation. Research Network on SES and Health. Available at http://www.macses.ucsf.edu. Accessed 1/3/2013.

Martz, E., and H. Livneh. *Coping with Chronic Illness and Disability: Theoretical, Empirical, and Clinical Aspects*. New York: Springer, 2007.

Marucha, P. T., J. K. Kiecolt-Glaser, and M. Favagehi. "Mucosal Wound Healing Is Impaired by Examination Stress." *Psychosomatic Medicine* 60, no. 3 (1998): 362–365.

Marx, D. M., S. J. Ko, and R. Friedman. "The 'Obama Effect': How a Salient Role Model Reduces Race-Based Performance Differences." *Journal of Experimental Psychology* 45 (2009): 953–956.

Maslach, C. *The Truth about Burnout: How Organizations Cause Personal Stress and What to Do about It.* San Francisco, CA: Jossey-Bass, 1997.

Mayer, J. D., P. Salovey, and D. Caruso. "Models of Emotional Intelligence." In Sternberg, R. (ed.) *Handbook of Intelligence* (pp. 396–420). Cambridge, UK: Cambridge University Press, 2000.

McEwen, B. S. "Stress, Adaptation, and Disease: Allostasis and Allostatic Load." *Annals of the New York Academy of Sciences* 840 (May 1, 1998): 33–44.

McGinnis, J. M., P. G. Ruso, and J. R. Knickman. "The Case for More Active Policy Attention to Health Promotion." *Health Affairs* 21, no. 2 (2002): 78–93.

McGonigal, K. *The Willpower Instinct: How Self-Control Works, Why It Matters, and How You Can Get More of It.* New York: Penguin Books, 2012.

McKay, M., P. D. Rogers, and J. McKay. *When Anger Hurts: Quieting the Storm Within.* 2nd ed. San Francisco, CA: New Harbinger, 2003.

Miller, W. R., and C. E. Thoresen. "Spirituality, Religion, and Health: An Emerging Research Field." *American Psychologist* 58, no.1 (2003): 24–35.

Miller, W. R., and S. Rollnick. *Motivational Interviewing: Preparing People for Change.* 2nd ed. New York, NY: Guilford Press, 2002.

Morin, C. M., C. Colecchi, J. Stone, R. Sood, and D. Brink. "Behavioral and Pharmacological Therapies for Late-Life Insomnia: A Randomized Controlled Trial." *Journal of the American Medical Association* 281, 11 (1999): 991–999.

Nuon, P. "Phaly's Story." Available at http://www.eglobalfamily.org/phaly-story.html. Accessed 1/11/2013.

Paul, A. M. *Origins: How the Nine Months before Birth Shape the Rest of Our Lives.* New York: Free Press, 2010.

Pennebaker, J. *Opening Up: The Healing Power of Expressing Emotions.* New York: Guilford Press, 1997.

Prochaska, J. O., J. C. Norcross, and C. C. DiClemente. *Changing for Good.* New York: Avon Books, 1994.

Reivich, K., and A. Shatte. *The Resilience Factor: 7 Keys to Finding Your Inner Strength and Overcoming Life's Hurdles.* New York: Broadway Publishing, 2002.

Remen, R. *Kitchen Table Wisdom: Stories That Heal.* New York: Berekeley Publishing Group, 1996.

Rollnick, S., P. Mason, and C. Butler. *Health Behavior Change: A Guide for Practitioners.* New York: Churchill Livingstone, 2000.

Rosen, M. *Thank You for Being Such a Pain: Spiritual Guidance for Dealing with Difficult People.* New York: Three Rivers Press, 1999.

Rothbaum, B., E. Foa, and E. Hembree. *Reclaiming Your Life from a Traumatic Experience: A Prolonged Exposure Treatment Program Workbook.* New York: Oxford University Press, 2007.

Salzberg, S. *Loving-Kindness: The Revolutionary Art of Happiness.* Rev. ed. Boston, MA: Shambhala Publications, Inc., 2002.

Sapolsky, R. *Why Zebras Don't Get Ulcers*. New York: Holt Paperbacks, 2004.

Satterfield, J. M. *A Cognitive-Behavioral Approach to the Beginning of the End of Life: Minding the Body*. New York: Oxford University Press, 2008.

———. *Minding the Body: Workbook*. New York: Oxford University Press, 2008.

Schattner, A. "The Silent Dimension: Expressing Humanism in Each Medical Encounter." *Archives of Internal Medicine* 169, no.12 (June 22, 2009): 1095–1099.

Schimpff, S. C. *The Future of Medicine: Megatrends in Healthcare That Will Improve Your Quality of Life*. Nashville, TN: Thomas Nelson, 2007.

Scott, J. "Life at the Top in America Isn't Just Better, It's Longer: Three Heart Attacks and What Came Next." *The New York Times*. May 16, 2005.

Seligman, M. E. P. *Authentic Happiness: Using the New Positive Psychology to Realize Your Potential for Lasting Fulfillment*. New York: Free Press, 2004.

———. *Flourish: A Visionary New Understanding of Happiness and Well-Being*. New York: Free Press, 2012.

———. *Learned Optimism*. New York: Alfred Knopf, 1991.

Snyder, C. R. *Coping: The Psychology of What Works*. New York: Oxford University Press, 1999.

Solomon, A. *The Noonday Demon: An Atlas of Depression*. New York: Touchstone, 2002.

Spector, M. "Germs Are Us: Bacteria Make Us Sick. Do They Also Keep Us Alive?" *The New Yorker*. Oct. 22, 2012.

Spiegel, D., J. R. Bloom, H. C. Kraemer, and E. Gottheil. "Effect of Psychosocial Treatment on Survival of Patients with Metastatic Breast Cancer." *The Lancet* 334, 8668 (October 14, 1989): 888–891.

Steele, C. M., and J. Aronson. "Stereotype Threat and the Intellectual Test Performance of African-Americans." *Journal of Personality and Social Psychology* 69 (1995): 797–811.

Stone, J., C. Lynch, M. Sjomeling, and J. M. Darley. "Stereotype Threat Effects on Black and White Athletic Performance." *Journal of Personality and Social Psychology* 77 (1999): 1213–1227.

Taylor, J. B. *My Stroke of Insight: A Brain Scientist's Personal Journey*. New York: Viking, 2008.

Thaler, R. H., and C. R. Sunstein. *Nudge: Improving Decisions about Health, Wealth, and Happiness*. New Haven, CT: Yale University Press, 2008.

Thompson, T. *The Beast: A Journey through Depression*. New York: Plume, 1996.

Tollefsbol, T. *Epigenetics in Human Disease*. Waltham, MA: Academic Press, 2012.

Topol, E. *The Creative Destruction of Medicine: How the Digital Revolution Will Create Better Healthcare*. New York: Basic Books, 2012.

Uchino, B. *Social Support and Physical Health: Understanding the Health Consequences of Relationships*. New Haven, CT: Yale University Press, 2004.

Ulrich, R. S. "View through a Window May Influence Recovery from Surgery." *Science* 224 (1984): 420–421.

U.S. Department of Health and Human Services. Office of Disease Prevention and Health Promotion. Healthy People 2020. Washington, DC. Available at http://www.healthypeople.gov/2020/default.aspx. Accessed 1/2/2013.

Valliant, G. *The Wisdom of the Ego*. Cambridge, MA: Harvard University Press, 1998.

World Health Organization. Top Ten Causes of Death. Available at http://www.who.int/mediacentre/factsheets/fs310/en/index.html. Accessed 1/3/2013.

Notes

Notes

Notes